Play Therapy Today

Play Therapy Today brings together the work of renowned practitioners and academics currently working and researching in therapeutic play and play therapy, and presents a range of ground-breaking methods for practising with groups, individuals, parents and carers.

Providing an overview of new or revitalised topics in play therapy, each chapter presents the relevant theoretical underpinnings and principles of practice, a guide to implementing the method and case study vignettes of the approach in practice. The three sections include chapters on:

- The therapeutic touchstone model and the development of the therapeutic relationship, an overview of the use of individual play therapy techniques with children in a hospital setting, and an overview of Yasenik and Gardner's Play Therapy Dimensions Model with an in-depth exploration of the dimension of consciousness from both a theoretical and practical, play-based orientation.
- Jennings' Embodiment-Project-Role model and its implementation in group work, the practical use of puppets in educational and therapeutic settings, the therapeutic value of working with groups in the outdoors, and the use of play in groups for children with a variety of sensory, intellectual and physical disabilities.
- Stagnitti's adaptation of the 'Learn to Play' programme for parent/carer use, Theraplay® with peer groups and parent/child dyads and how a neurosequential approach supports case conceptualization and play therapy practice with families.

The book provides practitioners with up-to-date, effective and practical techniques that they can put into immediate use in their clinical work with children and their families. It is an important resource for trainee, newly qualified and seasoned play therapists, play therapy supervisors and trainers. It will also be of interest to social workers, teachers, psychologists, child psychotherapists and other health professionals.

Eileen Prendiville is a Course Director at the Children's Therapy Centre in Co. Westmeath, Ireland. Eileen has worked with children for over 35 years and now specialises in the field of play therapy training. She was a founder member of the Children at Risk in Ireland Foundation and was their National Clinical Director until 2004. She is the current Chairperson of the Irish Association of Humanistic and Integrative Psychotherapy.

Justine Howard is an Associate Professor and Postgraduate Programme Manager at the Centre for Children and Young People's Health and Wellbeing at Swansea University, UK. She is a Chartered Psychologist and specialist in Developmental and Therapeutic Play.

'A comprehensive presentation of current practices in the field of Play Therapy. Highly recommended!'
– *Charles E. Schaefer, PhD, RPT-S, Cofounder & Director Emeritus, the Association for Play Therapy*

'What a wonderful new addition to our field! Each chapter is authored by an experienced clinician and expert in the topic and it clearly shows. It is refreshing to read clearly articulated approaches with case examples. The result is the ability to easily put the information into action. In fact, I used two of the techniques right away with current clients. Another chapter assisted me in viewing a client in a new way, assisting to facilitate more effective treatment. What a delight. I believe this book will be found valuable by both the new and seasoned play therapist.'
– *Linda E. Homeyer, PhD, RPT-S, Professor, Texas State University, USA*

Play Therapy Today

Contemporary practice with individuals, groups and carers

Edited by Eileen Prendiville and Justine Howard

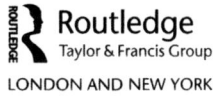

LONDON AND NEW YORK

First published 2014
by Routledge
2 Park Square, Milton Park, Abingdon, Oxon, OX14 4RN

and by Routledge
711 Third Avenue, New York, NY 10017

Routledge is an imprint of the Taylor & Francis Group, an informa business

© 2014 selection and editorial material, Eileen Prendiville and Justine Howard; individual chapters, the contributors

The right of the editors to be identified as the authors of the editorial material, and of the authors for their individual chapters, has been asserted in accordance with sections 77 and 78 of the Copyright, Designs and Patents Act 1988.

All rights reserved. No part of this book may be reprinted or reproduced or utilised in any form or by any electronic, mechanical, or other means, now known or hereafter invented, including photocopying and recording, or in any information storage or retrieval system, without permission in writing from the publishers.

Trademark notice: Product or corporate names may be trademarks or registered trademarks, and are used only for identification and explanation without intent to infringe.

British Library Cataloguing in Publication Data
A catalogue record for this book is available from the British Library

Library of Congress Cataloging-in-Publication Data
Play therapy today : contemporary practice with individuals, groups, and carers / edited by Eileen Prendiville and Justine Howard.
p. ; cm.
Includes bibliographical references.
I. Prendiville, Eileen, 1958- editor of compilation. II. Howard, Justine, editor of compilation.
[DNLM: 1. Child. 2. Play Therapy–methods. 3. Child Psychology. 4. Models, Theoretical. WS 350.4]
RJ505.P6
618.92'891653–dc23
2013044399

ISBN: 978-0-415-85505-1 (hbk)
ISBN: 978-0-415-85506-8 (pbk)
ISBN: 978-0-203-74028-6 (ebk)

Typeset in Sabon
by Cenveo Publisher Services

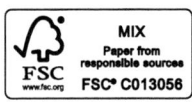

Printed and bound in Great Britain by
TJ International Ltd, Padstow, Cornwall

With an abundance of love to my granddaughter, Emilia

You are an amazing baby girl and I am so excited about the wonderful opportunity I have for close-up play and laughter with you throughout your lifetime. I have such delightful memories of playing with your mum, Siobhán, and your uncles Oisin and Cian. How wonderful to see my baby girl with her baby girl – the cycle continues!

Eileen

Contents

List of figures and tables	ix
Contributor biographies	x
Foreword by Dr Athena Drewes	xv
Introduction	1

SECTION I
Using play therapeutically with individual clients   5

1   The therapeutic touchstone   7
 EILEEN PRENDIVILLE

2   The consciousness dimension in play therapy: sharpening the play therapist's focus and skills   29
 LORRI YASENIK AND KEN GARDNER

3   Using play therapeutically with children in a hospital setting   47
 LISA MORGAN AND JUSTINE HOWARD

4   Therapeutic play as an intervention for children exposed to domestic violence   64
 TRISH GETTINS

SECTION II
Using play therapeutically with groups   79

5   Applying an Embodiment-Projection-Role framework
in groupwork with children   81
SUE JENNINGS

6   The use of puppets in therapeutic and educational settings   97
SIOBHÁN PRENDIVILLE

7   Working therapeutically with groups in the outdoors:
a natural space for healing   113
MAGGIE FEARN

8   Group play therapy for children with multiple disabilities   130
EIMIR MCGRATH

SECTION III
Using play therapeutically with parents and carers   147

9   The *Parent Learn to Play* program: building relationships
through play   149
KAREN STAGNITTI

10   Group Theraplay®   163
EVANGELINE MUNNS

11   How neuroscience can inform play therapy practice
with parents and carers   179
THERESA FRASER

Index   199

List of figures and tables

Figures

1.1	Maslow's hierarchy of needs diagram	24
2.1	Play Therapy Dimensions diagram	31
3.1	Play specialist using the puppet, Boris, with a child	54
3.2	Example of a completed dream sheet picture	56
3.3	Example of a dream sheet story	57
5.1	Picture of *Goldilocks and the Three Bears* by Charlie Meyer	93

Tables

3.1	Example of a structured play timetable	50
4.1	The impact of exposure to domestic abuse across developmental domains	67
9.1	Content and underpinning skills of the *Parent Learn to Play* program	154
11.1	A neurodevelopmental approach to case conceptualization and treatment planning	191

Contributor biographies

Editors

Eileen Prendiville is the Course Director for the MA in Humanistic & Integrative Psychotherapy and Play Therapy, the Postgraduate Diploma in Play Therapy and the Diploma in Child Psychotherapy and Play Therapy, at the Children's Therapy Centre in Co. Westmeath, Ireland. Eileen has worked with children for over 35 years and now specialises in the field of play therapy training. She has trained and worked in the fields of pre-school education, intellectual disability and child psychiatry; she has particular expertise in working with issues of child sexual abuse. Eileen holds qualifications in Humanistic and Integrative Psychotherapy, Jungian Sand Play Therapy, Biodynamic Psychotherapy and Family Law. She was a founder member of the Children at Risk in Ireland Foundation and was their National Clinical Director until 2004. She is a psychotherapist, play therapist, supervisor and teacher. She is the current Chairperson of the Irish Association of Humanistic and Integrative Psychotherapy. She has a chapter on 'Abreaction' in the 2nd edition of Dr Charles Schaefer's seminal text, *The Therapeutic Powers of Play: 20 Core Agents of Change*, co-authored with Dr Athena Drewes.

Justine Howard, PhD, CPsychol, AFBPsS, is an Associate Professor and Postgraduate Programme Manager at the Centre for Children and Young Peoples' Health and Wellbeing at Swansea University, UK. She is a Chartered Psychologist and specialist in Developmental and Therapeutic Play. She has wide ranging classroom experience in primary schools and worked for a number of years alongside children with additional learning needs, before training as a psychologist. She has been researching play and teaching developmental and educational psychology in higher education for over a decade. Her consultancy activity has included the delivery of training courses in developmental and therapeutic play for a wide range of professionals in children's services. She has published a number of journal articles, book chapters and books in the field of play and is regularly asked to speak at national and international conferences. Her most recent books include *The Essence of Play* (2013) and *Play in Early Childhood from Birth to Three Years* (2010).

Chapter contributors

Maggie Fearn, MA (Developmental and Therapeutic Play), has been a play practitioner for 30 years and a Forest School practitioner since 2001. She facilitates play sessions with children and young people of all ages and abilities in Wales, and she trains adults in non-directive play skills. She is also a graduate teacher of Body and Earth, experiential anatomy, somatics and authentic movement. In 2009 she completed an MA with distinction in Developmental and Therapeutic Play. Her research looked at nonverbal communication behaviour between mothers and children under 3 years during outdoor play. She is in demand as a speaker about the therapeutic value of outdoor play, and the importance of attending to children's perspectives. In 2011 she co-founded Movement Sense, a community interest company established to manage and develop places, spaces and experiences for individuals, groups and communities to access and engage with the natural environment for wellbeing, learning and creative expression through the moving body.

Theresa Fraser has worked with children and youth since 1983. She and her husband have been Treatment foster parents since 1990. She is the current President of the Canadian Association for Child and Play Therapy, a Play Therapy Supervisor and has specialized in working with children who have trauma and attachment disruptions for most of her career. She also is a Professor in the Child and Youth Worker program at Sheridan College in Ontario, Canada and has written two books, *Billy Had to Move: A Foster Care Story* and *Adopting a Child with a Trauma and Attachment Disruption History*, as well as many articles and book chapters.

Ken Gardner, MSc, RPsych, CPT-S, is a Clinical Psychologist and certified play therapy supervisor with 25 years of counselling experience. Through the Rocky Mountain Play Therapy Institute, Ken has presented nationally and internationally on a wide range of topics related to play therapy and supervision. Ken has served as an executive board member on the Canadian Association for Child and Play Therapy. His specializations include play-based interventions for children with developmental challenges, achievement motivation, and assessment and interventions for children with learning difficulties.

Trish Gettins completed her Masters in Developmental and Therapeutic Play at the College of Human Health Science, Swansea University, UK. During this time she focused her thesis on interventions to support the emotional health of children affected by domestic violence. Her research was well received and initiated a successful career working for Women's Aid in Wales. Trish helped to develop their dedicated children and young persons project as a therapeutic play specialist. Trish has presented at the International Play Association Conference and Respect Conference sharing best practice. Trish is about to embark on a new adventure as a play specialist to help develop a new project in Qatar within a women and children's hospital.

Sue Jennings, PhD, is Honorary Fellow at Leeds Metropolitan, and Roehampton Universities. She is a Play and Dramatherapist and Storyteller. Her early play therapy practice, from the mid-80s, developed a groupwork model for working with young children and families; her play research has focused on exploring the dramatic impulse in infants and children, and its relevance cross-culturally in understanding child development. More recently she has pioneered Neuro-Dramatic-Play. She works in Romania and Malaysia, where she conducted her doctoral fieldwork with the Temiar peoples in the Malaysian rainforest. She is a prolific author, and a Churchill Fellow 2012–2013.

Eimir McGrath, PhD, is a psychotherapist specializing in play therapy, as well as lecturing and teaching in several disciplines including play therapy, disability studies and dance. She has worked in a wide variety of educational and clinical settings and has extensive experience in working therapeutically with children and adults with disabilities. She has recently completed her doctoral studies; the intersection of psychotherapy, dance and critical disability studies provided the basis for her research, which focused on interpersonal neurobiology and dance performance as a means of challenging disablism. She has contributed a chapter to *Disability and Social Theory: New Developments and Directions* published by Palgrave McMillan in 2012. She is a play therapy trainer at the Children's Therapy Centre in Co. Westmeath, Ireland.

Lisa Morgan originally qualified as a nursery nurse and for a number of years worked alongside children aged 4–7 years in a primary school environment. For the past 17 years she has worked as a nursery nurse and play specialist on a busy paediatric surgical ward at Morriston Hospital in Swansea, UK. Her role involves utilizing a variety of therapeutic play techniques in pre- and post-operative care – in particular, distraction techniques, puppets, storytelling and guided imagery. She has lectured about the therapeutic value of play in hospital settings at postgraduate level and is currently completing an MA in Developmental and Therapeutic Play at Swansea University, UK.

Evangeline Munns, PhD, CPsych, RPT-S, CTT-S., CACPT-S, is a certified clinical psychologist with over 40 years of experience working with troubled children and their parents. She was the former clinical director of Play Therapy Services at Blue Hills Child and Family Centre in Aurora, Ontario in Canada, which under her leadership became the largest training school in Theraplay in Canada. Evangeline is a certified therapist, supervisor and trainer with the Theraplay® Institute, the Association of Play Therapy in the US and the Canadian Association of Play Therapy. From the latter she received the Monica Herbert award for 'an outstanding contribution to the field of play therapy in Canada'. Evangeline is a popular presenter throughout Canada, the United States and internationally. She mainly spends her time teaching, supervising, consulting and writing.

Siobhán Prendiville, BEd, PGEd, MEd, Diploma Play Therapy and Psychotherapy, is a teacher and play therapist who specializes in the use of play in education and in therapy. She received her play therapy and psychotherapy qualifications at the Children's Therapy Centre in Co. Westmeath, Ireland. Her main research interests are in the developmental and therapeutic use of puppets, sand, and water play. She teaches widely in a number of institutions in Ireland and is involved in training teachers in pilot programmes to influence the teaching methodologies utilized. In addition to her teaching positions, she maintains a private play therapy practice. Siobhán has a chapter on 'Accelerated Psychological Development' in the 2nd edition of Dr Charles Schaefer's seminal text, *The Therapeutic Powers of Play: 20 Core Agents of Change*, co-authored with Dr Athena Drewes.

Karen Stagnitti currently works as Professor, Personal Chair, at the School of Health and Social Development at Deakin University, Victoria, Australia. Over the past 30+ years she has mainly worked in early childhood intervention programmes in community-based settings as part of a specialist, paediatric multidisciplinary team. In 2003 she graduated from LaTrobe University with a Doctor of Philosophy. Her area of research is children's play. Karen has written numerous books and book chapters on play and has over 60 national and international papers published. Her norm-referenced standardized play assessment, the Child-Initiated Pretend Play Assessment has been used in several research studies to examine: relationships between pretend play, language and social skills; social-emotional understanding and play complexity; play ability in children with autism spectrum disorder; and abilities of children who attend different types of school curriculum. She developed the Learn to Play programme for children with developmental difficulties who did not have play skills. This programme is now used in several countries.

Lorri Yasenik, PhD, MSW, RPT-S, CPT-S, is a Co-Director of Rocky Mountain Play Therapy Institute in Calgary Alberta, Canada. Lorri is the co-author of the *Play Therapy Dimensions Model: A Decision-Making Model for Integrative Play Therapists* (2012) as well as book chapters on play therapy supervision and play therapy techniques. Lorri is a certified and registered play therapist supervisor and a founding member of Alberta Play Therapy Association. She trains nationally and internationally in the areas of play therapy, child psychotherapy, attachment, trauma and high conflict separation and divorce.

Foreword

Athena A. Drewes, PsyD, RPT-S

Just as birds fly and fish swim, children play (Landreth, 2002). It is as natural as breathing for them. Through the use of toys they find voice in expressing their inner world through their play. Horrific images can be expressed, past traumas revisited in the safe space of the therapy room with an empathic play therapist. Healing can begin to happen.

Play is not just a medium or context for applying other interventions; inherent within play behaviours is a broad spectrum of active forces that produce behaviour change (Schaefer and Drewes, 2014). In essence, healing and therapeutic powers exist in play.

Therapeutic powers transcend culture, language, age and gender. Therapeutic powers of play refers to the specific change agents in which play initiates, facilitates or strengthens their therapeutic effect. Thus play actually helps produce the change and is not just a medium for applying other change agents, nor does it just moderate the strength or direction of the therapeutic change. Schaefer and Drewes (2014) identified 20 core therapeutic powers of play. Play, the child's natural language, is often the easiest way for children to express troubling thoughts and feelings that are both conscious and unconscious. And by making learning an enjoyable experience, therapists are best able to impart the information needed by clients to overcome knowledge and skills deficits. Powers that help to facilitate communication include: self-expression; access to the unconscious; direct teaching; and indirect teaching (Schaefer and Drewes, 2014).

In order to develop better awareness of and control over distressing feelings, play helps to strengthen the emotional health and well-being of our child clients. Powers of play that foster emotional wellness include catharsis, abreaction, positive emotions, counter-conditioning fears, stress inoculation and stress management (Schaefer and Drewes, 2014).

Beginning in infancy, the stages of sensory-motor, construction, pretend and game play promote social development by triggering feelings of attachment, warmth, empathy and respect for others. Therapeutic powers of play that enhance social relationships include therapeutic relationship, attachment, social competence and empathy (Schaefer and Drewes, 2014).

Finally, play has been found to foster an array of personal strengths that help clients overcome both internal weaknesses and external stressors. Play, in particular, can boost a child's development, self-control, self-esteem, creativity, and resiliency. Therapeutic powers of play that increase personal strengths include creative problem solving, resiliency, moral development, accelerated psychological development, self-regulation and self-esteem (Schaefer and Drewes, 2014).

In order to be the best therapist possible, we need a full arsenal of the therapeutic powers of play to effectively and efficiently overcome the many forces of psychopathology.

Eileen Prendiville and Justine Howard offer us an arsenal of ways to use the therapeutic powers of play in *Play Therapy Today: Contemporary practice with individuals, groups and carers.* This composite of eleven chapters by renowned play therapists in England, Ireland, Australia and Canada covers an array of topics, techniques and practical applications that will enhance play therapy treatment with children and families.

Section 1: Using play therapeutically with individual clients opens with Eileen Prendiville's chapter outlining her 'Therapeutic Touchstone' approach that facilitates the development of the therapeutic relationship through being authentic, open, honest and clear from the first meeting. The goal of creating a therapeutic story as to why the child has come for therapy is laid out in a step-wise fashion for immediate application by the reader in the initial stages of treatment. Lorri Yasenik and Ken Gardner follow with 'The consciousness dimension in play therapy: sharpening the play therapist's focus and skills'. This integrative, decision-making model helps to focus the therapist's intentionality and thoughtfulness in attending during play activities. 'Using play therapeutically with children in a hospital setting' by Lisa Morgan and Justine Howard follows and offers powerful case studies and examples on how best to use play therapeutically to enable children to gain a sense of autonomy and control in potentially distressing and unfamiliar situations. This section closes with 'Therapeutic play as an intervention for children exposed to domestic violence' by Trish Gettins. The author offers the reader specific ways in which the therapeutic powers of play work to increase resilience and emotional health in children, thereby helping to mediate the impact of exposure to domestic violence.

Section 2: Using Play therapeutically with groups opens with 'Applying an Embodiment-Projection-Role framework in groupwork with children' by Sue Jennings. Children's creative play process and the facilitation of social and emotional growth is enhanced through use of NDP and EPR. The reader is walked through the Neuro-Dramatic-Play (NDP) process and how Embodiment-Projection-Role (EPR) can enrich children, especially those struggling with communication, behaviour and attachment difficulties, to enhance their personal and social strengths through creative and therapeutic groupwork. This chapter is followed by Siobhán Prendiville's 'The use of puppets in therapeutic and educational settings'. We learn in detail how the magic and therapeutic use of puppets allows the child to project their inner thoughts and feelings onto puppets, thereby facilitating affective expression. Case examples and clear guidance give the inexperienced or unsure clinician support in using puppets. 'Working therapeutically with groups in the outdoors: a natural space for healing' by Maggie Fearn helps clinicians utilize, in groups, the therapeutic benefits of sensory exposure to nature for building attachment and self-regulation. This section closes with Eimir McGrath's chapter 'Group play therapy for children with multiple disabilities'. The therapeutic powers of social connection and relatedness, along with self-esteem, are enhanced through groupwork that focuses on rhythm, music and movement. Practical applications for children with disabilities are shared, enriching this chapter's usefulness for the reader.

Finally, **Section 3: Using play therapeutically with parents and carers** offers readers three chapters devoted to working on building attachment and relationships, thereby helping to reduce the negative impact that adverse experiences have had on the brain development of the child.

Karen Stagnitti begins with 'The *Parent Learn to Play* programme: building relationships through play', a comprehensive 24-week programme that builds 12 skills through the use of pretend play between children as developmentally young as 12–18 months and the parent or carer, thereby enhancing attachment. Evangeline Munns follows with 'Group Theraplay®' utilizing the therapeutic power of touch to create and enhance attachment, whilst also raising the self-esteem and confidence of the group participants.

Theresa Fraser ends the book with 'How neuroscience can inform play therapy practice with parents and carers'. This chapter helps the reader develop a deeper understanding of the impact of neglect and trauma on a child's developing brain and the use of a neurosequential model for remediation and intervention.

The clinician reading this book will find its strength lies in the many detailed practical approaches and programmes along with the case studies and examples. Each chapter will help to enrich your practice in play therapy with children and families. A book well worth keeping handy for constant reference!

References

Landreth, G. (2002). *Play Therapy: The Art of the Relationship* (2nd edn). Philadelphia, PA: Brunner/Routledge.
Schaefer, C. E. and Drewes, A. A. (2014). *The Therapeutic Powers of Play: 20 Core Agents of Change* (2nd edn). Hoboken, NJ: Wiley & Sons.

Athena A. Drewes, PsyD, MA, RPT-S, is the Director of Clinical Training and the APA-Accredited Internship at Astor Services for Children & Families, a multiservice non-profit agency in New York. She is past director of the Association for Play Therapy and serves on the editorial board of the *International Journal of Play Therapy*.

Introduction

Justine Howard

Eileen and I first met when I enrolled to train in developmental and therapeutic play at her Children's Therapy Centre in Ireland. My initial professional background was in primary education and behavioural support. I later trained in psychology and completed my PhD on play within the early years curriculum. From this stemmed an academic career in psychology, focusing primarily on evidencing the beneficial effects of play for children across developmental domains. Through my professional practice and research I became interested in the therapeutic value of play and wished to extend my training in this area. Having been involved in empirical research into the benefits of play for over ten years as a psychologist, throughout the experiential training I felt compelled to critically evaluate the evidence upon which the practice being presented was based. I am certain that both Eileen and Sue Jennings, as the trainers at the time, will remember my constant stream of annoying questions! However, the discussions which ensued during my visits to the Centre between the trainers and the other students were illuminating.

Whilst the group of students came from a variety of different backgrounds (hospital play, playwork, social work, counselling, education, psychotherapy, dramatherapy and play therapy), the foundations that underpinned effective professional practice were relevant to each of us. Axline's play therapy principles, key playwork approaches and the effective use of play in early years classrooms, hospitals, and child welfare services all rely on empowering children, enabling them to govern their own play choices, retaining autonomy and control. We were also united in the belief that children's emotional health is at the heart of their development across domains. One of the difficulties in identifying such commonalities is that research findings and the resulting knowledge base which underpins our work have tended not to be shared across disciplines or areas of professional practice (Howard and McInnes, 2013).

I guess the reasons for this are not hard to explain. Play therapists have published their research findings in play therapy journals, educators in education journals, hospital play professionals in journals relating to nursing or health care and so on. However, with our increased understanding and acceptance of the power of play for supporting children's development, the practice of children's service professionals can no longer be pigeonholed. For example, we have seen a rise in emotional literacy programmes in primary schools. Children's emotional health, as well as their medical needs, is now central to paediatric hospital provision. The power of play is such that it is also not possible to have learning through play occurring only in school and healing through play occurring only in the therapy room. I have recently been working on a project focused on children's conversations and spontaneous play following natural disasters. The conversations and play were not recorded through counselling or therapy sessions but from children's day to day interactions in the school environment. This work highlighted the invaluable role of educators in facilitating therapeutic play and enabling children to talk about their earthquake experiences (Bateman *et al.* 2013).

It was only in 2012 that we saw the launch of the International Journal of Play, the first inter-disciplinary publication focusing on play theory, policy and practice from multiple perspectives. Since its launch, the range of topics covered in the journal has been extensive, including the challenge of integrating play into the early years curriculum; facilitating effective play environments; the value of play for children facing differences of diversity; cultural and historical perspectives on play; play and development across domains; and play with digital technologies.

The important role of an inter-disciplinary publication such as this is highlighted in the editor's reflections on the journal's first year. Broadhead (2013) talks of how one consistent challenge for the provision of effective practice is ensuring that children retain control over their play activity. Whether play is 'limited' or 'facilitated' depends on planning and legislation, characteristics of the environment and material provision, but perhaps, most importantly, a skilled play workforce. The skill of the adult in providing for children's optimum play experiences is largely dependent on their sensitivity to ensuring children's continued sense of autonomy and control.

Research clearly demonstrates that the autonomy and control children perceive over their play activities has a direct impact on their sense of playfulness (Robson, 1993; Keating *et al.* 2000; Howard, 2002). It is this playful disposition which separates play from the other types of activity in which children engage and renders it such a valuable mechanism for learning and development across domains. As my colleague and I have written elsewhere, there are particular benefits of playfulness that are now well evidenced from research across a range of disciplines: playfulness promotes the development or restoration of attachment bonds and other social relationships; it provides a means of effective communication; promotes children's independence and self-regulation; enhances confidence and esteem; provides strategies for dealing with conflict and anxiety; promotes flexible and adaptive thinking skills; and leads to high levels of motivation and engagement (Howard and McInnes, 2013). When children are in control of their play, they are free to set and alter their own challenges and goals. This minimises feelings of failure, protects children's sense of self and promotes emotional wellbeing. As such, play supports resiliency (Fearn and Howard, 2011) and acts as a resource that enables children to meet the physical, intellectual and emotional challenges of their daily lives (Howard, 2010).

I hope that you will enjoy reading this book as much as Eileen and I have enjoyed its editing and compilation. It contains chapters from experienced practitioners and researchers working across a range of children's service contexts. The chapters, eloquently summarised by Athena in her Foreword, capture the power of play for working with groups, individual children and their families and carers. Each author demonstrates the importance of play for supporting children's emotional health but also, like the conversations which took place during my training, the book as a whole highlights the threads of thinking that unify us as play professionals.

Note

Throughout the book, the names of healthcare practitioners who were interviewed and children who appear within case studies have been changed or omitted for confidentiality reasons.

References

Bateman, A., Danby, S. and Howard, J. (2013). Everyday preschool talk about Christchurch earthquakes. *Australian Journal of Communication*, 40 (1), 103–122.

Broadhead, P. (2013). Looking back over the first year of the International Journal of Play. *International Journal of Play*, 2 (1), 1–3.

Fearn, M. and Howard, J. (2011). Play as a resource for children facing adversity: An exploration of indicative case studies. *Children and Society*, doi: 10.1111/j.1099-0860.2011.00357.

Howard, J. (2002). Eliciting young children's perceptions of play, work and learning using the activity apperception story procedure. *Early Child Development and Care*, 172, 489–502.

Howard, J. (2010). The developmental and therapeutic potential of play: re-establishing teachers as play professionals. In J. Moyles (ed.), *The Excellence of Play* (3rd edn), (pp 201–215) Maidenhead: Open University Press.

Howard, J. and McInnes, K. (2013). *The Essence of Play: A practice companion for professionals working with children and young people.* London: Routledge.

Keating, I., Fabian, H., Jordan, P., Mavers, D. and Roberts, J. (2000). 'Well, I've not done any work today. I don't know why I came to school'. Perceptions of play in the reception class. *Educational Studies*, 26 (4), 437–454.

Robson, S. (1993). 'Best of all I like choosing time': Talking with children about play and work. *Early Child Development and Care*, 92, 37–51.

1 Using play therapeutically with individual clients

1 The therapeutic touchstone

Eileen Prendiville

The therapeutic touchstone is a play-based intervention used to facilitate the development of a therapeutic relationship with children and adolescents. The therapist presents a synopsis of significant elements in the child's life story to the child, and their parents or other supportive ally, using toys to facilitate building the play therapy relationship. While it is a focused, directive, narrative intervention, it is based on Rogerian principles (Rogers, 1980). In this chapter I provide a rationale for this intervention and provide detailed guidelines for constructing and presenting these stories.

Rogers believed that if the therapist held certain *attitudes* toward the client, therapeutic change would occur: if the therapist truly believes and trusts that the client knows what is best for herself, and if the therapist embodies the identified attitudes, this will create the optimum environment for the client to grow and initiate change that brings them closer to self-actualization. Rogers identified what he believed to be the core conditions essential for facilitating this growth. In relation to the therapist, we generally refer to the 3 core conditions of unconditional positive regard, empathy and congruence. Rogers considered congruence as being essential in facilitating a real meeting between counsellor and client, to enable the client to experience something/somebody 'from the outside'. This is the attitude that is central in my touchstone stories. For me, being authentic with my child clients requires me to bring openness, honesty and clarity to our first meeting and this involves me letting them know, in an age appropriate way, what I already know about them and how I came to know it. This is the basis for my story-making approach.

According to one dictionary (http://www.thefreedictionary.com), a touchstone is an 'excellent quality or example that is used to test the excellence or genuineness of others'. When used as a noun it is 'a standard by which judgment is made'. Telling the child's story in a child friendly way following the touchstone technique in the first meeting enables the therapist to demonstrate genuineness, assisting the child in evaluating their openness, honesty and trustworthiness. Thus it is a starting point for developing a powerful therapeutic relationship and sets the context for the therapy process. Many children referred for play therapy have trust issues; we cannot expect them to trust us straight away. In fact, developing the ability to trust is often an end result rather than a starting point in therapy. We must demonstrate our trustworthiness in a developmentally appropriate way. It is not enough to simply allow the child to communicate in their language with us – we also need to communicate with them in that language. Therefore we need to use play, and playfulness, when we have something important to communicate to our young clients. For me, letting the child know what we know about them, and how we found out, is the first step in demonstrating trustworthiness.

The intake process

Before meeting a new child client, the play therapist will receive a referral, meet with carers, and consider relevant information, sometimes including reports, to enable them to assess the appropriateness of the referral, determine if they can offer the most appropriate services for the child at this time, and consider relevant issues in relation to the child's past, immediate future, and their current safety and protection. In this process there is the potential for the therapist to learn a lot about the child. Personally, I like to use the intake appointment with parents as an opportunity to explore their past and present experiences of their child and the problems they struggle with, to generate descriptions of positive aspects of the child's life, their personality, shared experiences, and to re-connect with parental hopes and positive emotions in relation to their child and their relationship. I hope to enable the parents to begin to separate the problems from the child. I want them to remember a time when the problems did not exist, or were not so severe, when they felt hopeful and connected to their child. For some parents this is easy, for others they may have moved to a place where they take the child's difficulties personally, may have lost sight of the child's struggle, and may experience the child as a very negative force in their lives. In taking this narrative approach, I am: gathering information to enrich my therapeutic touchstone story; enabling parents to reframe their current situation; building a solid framework for a working in partnership relationship; trying to generate hope for the future; helping parents to become more able to meet their child's needs; and acting as a supportive ally to their child during, and after, the psychotherapy process.

When a child comes to therapy, they are aware that the therapist already knows 'stuff' about them. They will also be aware that people in their world, perhaps including themselves, may want them to be different (or behave/feel differently). They may also have had difficult experiences that are linked to feelings of shame or guilt. The child may have been through an assessment in which they felt vulnerable or exposed. They may well be concerned that the therapist is judging them as being bad or shameful, or indeed they might fear the therapist if they have learned through previous experiences that adults can be dangerous or intrusive. There can also be a pressure on children entering therapy to tell the therapist about events (e.g. abuse, trauma) or symptoms (e.g. soiling, bullying) that they do not wish to discuss. This can contribute to high levels of anxiety and stress. As therapists we wish to establish the therapy room, and relationship, as being safe as soon as possible and this is where the therapeutic touchstone can help. It also helps in sowing seeds for the child to re-author their own experiences, to reframe difficulties, to externalize problems, and it provides the distance that will subsequently assist the child in reorganizing their personal identity.

Engaging the child

While there is a lot of content in the touchstone story, it is important to keep it short so as to hold the child's attention and help them manage whatever anxiety they might feel. This means that it should never take longer than six minutes to tell, less for children under six years of age (three minutes for a three-year-old, four for a four-year-old, and five for a five-year-old). The aim is to make it as attractive and engaging as possible. This means using play, and playfulness, rather than relying on words alone. The therapist tells this story while using miniature dolls and toys to dramatize it, so that the child, and her parents, can watch the play story being enacted as they listen. The dolls will have the same names as the family members and will, mostly, be referred to by these names rather than the therapist referring directly to the family members present for the session. Using play reduces the child's anxiety by providing dramatic distance from the content of the story. The therapist needs to be animated when presenting it, aiming to engage the child on a sensory and somatic level, and to create a picture, an externalized scene, with which the child can engage. Adding sound effects and using gestures, facial expressions and voice tone effectively is beneficial. Adding expressions such as 'Once upon a time' and contextualising it as being set 'in a land not too far from here' helps to provide dramatic distance, and assists in preventing the child from becoming overwhelmed. This is important as the story may refer to distressing life events, have emotionally laden content, and could make the child feel exposed if not carefully written and delivered. The therapist provides safety and facilitates active engagement by relying on:

> the psychological distance that is afforded by the use of metaphors and projections in the play process.... The 'as if' qualities of play allow for the duality of something being real and not real at the same time, allowing the child to take advantage of the emotional distancing, and safety, that is afforded by the use of symbols and metaphors.
> (Prendiville, 2014: 86–87).

Monitoring the child's reactions when telling the story

It is important to monitor the child's reactions when telling the story to ensure that the child does not become overwhelmed and that they are supported in staying regulated. The dramatic distance provided by using doll characters can facilitate this, however; because they identify with their own character in the story they will travel on the same journey with them – from calm beginnings, through the rough patches, and onto safer ground again. The therapist will utilize appropriate emotional tone throughout the storytelling experience. Through the action of mirror neurons, therapist-led regulatory interventions may become transformational experiences that contribute to neurobiological change (Levy, 2008) and enhance the child's ability to, for example, self-soothe and develop a coherent narrative.

Touchstone story structure for children with emotional/behavioural issues

The guidelines for preparing the story are linked to the level of complexity of the child's history. First, I am going to look at the guidelines for preparing the story for children who present with issues that are not known to be related to difficult life events; second, I will consider children with adjustment issues; and, third, address those with more complex histories. In this section, I am linking the guidelines to a sample story for a six-year-old child, Josie, where there are no known difficult life events that may have contributed to the presenting problems. It is not important to stick rigidly to this format – respond to the particular circumstances of each child.

1. Give the story a title.

    Josie and her sad and mad feelings

2. The beginning of the story is set at a stage before the presenting problems emerged. This is important as it reduces anxiety, allows the child to engage fully with the story, and reminds the family that there was a time when the current difficulties did not exist.

    Once upon a time, in a land not too far from here, a beautiful baby girl was born to parents who loved her very much. The parents' names were Jeff and Susan and they named their little girl Josie. She was so beautiful! Sometimes Jeff and Susan would just sit and stare at her with big, big smiles on their faces. They could hardly believe that she was real. (Continue to build profile of time before difficulties became evident.)

3. Show the emergence of the emotional or behavioural difficulties (including the presenting problems) and the response to these. Emphasize the presence of any secure attachments or supportive adults and include positive life experiences. Be aware that the child's anxiety may be provoked by references to presenting problems so be alert to any signs of distress and add elements that will be reassuring as indicated.

    Josie was a very popular girl and she had lots and lots of friends. But just before Christmas last year, when Josie was 5, Jeff and Susan began to notice that she did not want to play with her friends anymore, she wanted to be with Mummy and Daddy all the time. Sometimes she seemed very, very sad. Mummy and Daddy noticed that she would sit and rock, maybe sucking her thumb. Then she started to have temper tantrums like she had never had before. She would get so mad it was like there was a storm in the house. Everything would shake and sometimes it got very noisy. Mummy and Daddy hardly knew what to do. And sometimes Josie got into trouble in school too and the teacher would say, 'Tut, tut', shake her head and send Josie to the principal's office. Oh, what a lot of trouble!

    Sometimes when Josie would get upset Mummy would sit with her, take her on her knee and tell her how much she loved her. Sometimes they would have a lovely cuddle, but other times even this did not make Josie feel better. She would push Mummy away and say 'I hate you' or 'Leave me alone'. Other days it seemed like everything was OK again and the whole family would play in the garden, go to the park or even visit Granny and Grandad. Josie's friend, Emer, would came to play too and sometimes they would be happy together; other times they would fight and it would all end up in tears.

4. Refer to the current presence of a supportive ally. This reference will be in the wording of the story but the supportive ally will also be with the child during the telling of the story. Put emphasis on the carer's concern for the child rather than on dissatisfaction with his/her problematic behaviour.

   Mummy and Daddy were getting really worried. They wanted to sort this big mess out. They love Josie so much and want to be really sure that she is safe and they want to help her to find her happy heart again. They want to sort out any worries that Josie has and help her to play with her friends again in the ways that she used to.

5. Include the referral, intake sessions, and information that was made available to you. This section provides the opportunity to introduce the therapist and their work. Some therapists will also include references to confidentiality in the story at this point.

   So Mummy and Daddy had a chat and decided that something had to be done to help Josie. They heard about a lady called Eileen who plays with children in a special playroom, and guess what? When the children play here, they get to sort out their muddles and things get better! The children get to be the boss of playing and Eileen gets to be the boss of keeping everyone safe. There is just one big rule – the safe rule. That means that nobody gets hurt in the playroom and Eileen is in charge of that. Mummy and Daddy thought that this would be good for Josie so they went to see Eileen and told her all about the worries, about Josie being sad, not playing with her friends, and about the kicking and the shouting, too. Eileen explained that sometimes children act like that when they have very big feelings on the inside and they can't get them out any other way. She said that she could play with Josie to help her find new ways to let the feelings out. Eileen can also help Mummy and Daddy learn new ways to help Josie, too. Jeff was amazed when he heard that all Josie would have to do would be to play in lots of the ways that she wanted while she was in the playroom. Imagine that – playing to make things better!

6. Include references to the child's strengths and attractive qualities.

   Jeff and Susan know that Josie is really good at playing. They told Eileen that she loves puppets, playing with sand, drawing pictures, and especially making things out of playdough. They said that she is also very good at minding her puppy, and that she has a very sparkly smile. (I can see that now!!)

7. The story ends in the present tense – with the child attending the appointment and their story being told.

> *And that is how you all came to be here today, ready to see my playroom and start playing!*

Note that the story refers to the here and now when referring to the therapist and the playroom. The therapist stays focused on the play materials for most of the story, but also looks up, with a reassuring smile, to check in with the child and family at appropriate times (e.g. when speaking in present tense about the supportive ally, when seeing if Josie has a sparkly smile, when saying that playing makes things better). By linking directly with the family when presenting hope for the future and optimism about future positive change, the therapist communicates this confidence directly to the child and their carer/s.

Touchstone story structure for children with adjustment issues

When the child's difficulties are thought to be linked to distressing or confusing life experiences, or a difficulty in adjusting to a new situation, the story changes slightly.

Change from
1. Give the story a title.
2. The beginning of the story is set at a stage before the presenting problems emerged.
3. Show the emergence of the emotional or behavioural difficulties (including the presenting problems) and the response to these. Emphasize the presence of any secure attachments or supportive adults and do not ignore positive life experiences.

To
1. Give the story a title.
2. The beginning of the story is set at a stage before the difficult life event, emphasizes the presence of any secure attachments or supportive adults and includes positive life experiences.
3. Describe the difficult event briefly, using age appropriate language and show the emergence of the emotional or behavioural difficulties (including the presenting problems) and the response to these.
4. Continue as per previous list. . .

The story about Josie could be amended to the following.

This is a story about Josie and her sad and mad feelings.

Once upon a time, in a land not too far from here, a beautiful baby girl was born to parents who loved her very much. The parents' names were Jeff and Susan and they named their little girl Josie. She was so beautiful! Sometimes Jeff and Susan would just sit and stare at her with big, big smiles on their faces. They could hardly believe that she was real. (Continue to build profile of time before difficulties became evident.)

Josie was a very popular girl and she had lots and lots of friends. She had one very special friend called Sally who she loved very, very much. They played together nearly every day and sometimes had sleepovers. But then, just before Christmas last year, a really sad thing happened. Sally moved to a new house, far away. Josie missed her very, very much. Jeff and Susan began to notice that she did not want to play with her friends anymore; she wanted to be with Mummy and Daddy all the time. Sometimes she seemed very, very sad. Mummy and Daddy noticed that she would sit and rock, maybe sucking her thumb. Then she started to have temper tantrums like she had never had before. She would get so mad it was like there was a storm in the house. Everything would shake and sometimes it got very noisy. Mummy and Daddy hardly knew what to do. And sometimes Josie got into trouble in school too and the teacher would say, 'Tut, tut', shake her head and send Josie to the principal's office. Oh, what a lot of trouble!

Sometimes when Josie would get upset Mummy would sit with her, take her on her knee and tell her how much she loved her. Sometimes they would have a lovely cuddle, but other times even this did not make Josie feel better. She would push Mummy away and say, 'I hate you' or 'Leave me alone'. Other days it seemed like everything was OK again and the whole family would play in the garden, go to the park, or even visit Granny and Granddad. Josie's friend, Emer, would came to play too and sometimes they would be happy together; other times they would fight and it would all end up in tears.

Mummy and Daddy were getting really worried. They wanted to sort this big mess out. They love Josie so much and want to help her to find her happy heart again. They want to sort out any worries that Josie has and help her to play with her friends again in the ways that she used to.

So Mummy and Daddy had a chat and decided that something had to be done to help Josie. They heard about a lady called Eileen who plays with children in a special playroom, and guess what? When the children play here, they get to sort out their muddles and things get better! The children get to be the boss of playing and Eileen gets to be the boss of keeping everyone safe. There is just one big rule – the safe rule. That means that nobody gets hurt in the playroom and Eileen is in charge of that. Mummy and Daddy thought that this would be good for Josie so they went to see Eileen and told her all about Josie, what she used to like to do, about her being sad for a long time, not playing with her friends, and about the kicking and the shouting, too. Eileen explained that sometimes children act like that when they have very big feelings on the inside and they can't get them out any other way. She said that Josie must miss Sally very, very much and that maybe she was afraid that more people might go away. Susan told Eileen that there are no plans for anyone else to move. Eileen is going to help Mummy and Daddy learn new ways to help Josie. They made a plan to make a special book with photographs of Josie and Sally together, stories of the games they played together, and have arranged for a special visit to see Sally during the school holidays.

Eileen said that she could play with Josie to help her find new ways to let the feelings out. Jeff was amazed when he heard that all Josie would have to do would be to play in lots of the ways that she wanted while she was in the playroom. Imagine that – playing to make things better!

Jeff and Susan know that Josie is really good at playing. They told Eileen that she loves puppets, playing with sand, drawing pictures, and especially making things out of playdough. They said that she is also very good at minding her puppy, and that she has a very sparkly smile.

And that is how you all came to be here today, ready to see my playroom and start playing!

I believe that this technique provides a solid basis for working in a way that keeps the child's best interest as the paramount consideration at all times. It facilitates building the foundation for the play therapy relationship and is reassuring to the child as it removes a burden from them by communicating that we already know significant details of their experiences and difficulties and are still fully accepting of them.

Writing the touchstone story

Before writing the story the therapist needs to collect relevant information from the child's carers, and others involved in their world, and find appropriate wording to represent this adequately. Many referred children will have experienced disturbing events in their young lives. The therapist is interested in exploring any possible influences that may have contributed to the child's problematic mode of experiencing the world and themselves. They will make notes to highlight what they consider to be the most significant events and issues that may have caused the child to become confused and/or distressed. If there is a gap in the child's history, the therapist will try to find out more about that time in the child's life. If there is information missing that cannot be found, the gap may be referred to as part of the story.

Understanding the dynamics

The therapist will use their knowledge of associated dynamics to understand any complexities (for example, the grooming process, stages in bereavement, domestic violence, attachment, trauma). It is important to find child-friendly, age and stage appropriate, language to describe these issues and to enable the child to gain some understanding of their own experiences. Therapists are also advised to read therapeutic stories (e.g. Davis, 1985; Sunderland, 2000) to see how symbols and metaphors might be used to enhance the child's understanding of complex dynamics.

Each set of circumstances has to be considered carefully so that the wording matches the individual child's experiences. Do not try to copy exactly another person's examples, including those given here, as they will probably not match exactly with your client's needs. Some of the expressions I have used in touchstone stories are references to how the most important 'rules of the world' are about keeping children safe and that we know someone has broken these rules if a child gets hurt by someone touching them on a private part of the body and causes them to have mixed up, muddled feelings. Children who act out sexually can be described as having a 'touching problem'. Feelings of guilt and shame are directly addressed as many children will need particular assistance in overcoming these difficult emotions. In relation to pre-verbal memories, a child whose development was interrupted by early neglect or trauma, and who does not have memories of the events, might understand their difficulties more by hearing that 'when the thinking brain forgets, the body still remembers'. A child who experienced domestic violence and who put up a tough front really resonated with a story that described growing up in a house where there was 'lots of fighting and hurting' and how they 'felt sad on the inside' but learned not to show it on the outside. This was linked to a fear of how if you try not to pay attention to feeling hurt, you run the risk of 'closing your heart'. I have also made references to how a child's heart might be 'beating really fast, going boom, boom, boom, on the inside', how their 'tummy might be all wobbly', how they might be 'hardly able to breathe with the big fright they are getting', but they still manage 'to look all calm on the outside and even keep a big smile on their face'. Connecting with these somatic elements often intensifies how the child and their carers resonate with the story.

Repeated patterns in the child's life

If the child has a very complex history, do not try to give details of each change or event. Once the main theme has been presented, it is preferable to say something like 'lots of sad things happened', or that they lived in 'many different houses', rather than give a big list of every separate incident. You might find yourself making reference to something happening 'over and over again' if there has been chronic abuse or repeated incidents of trauma, or that 'everybody seemed to be going away' for a child who experienced multiple losses.

Other people's actions

It is also important to try to give some understanding of other peoples' actions in a way that will alleviate the responsibility that children often feel for the behaviour of others. A person might be described as having a 'heart that could not love', or a 'brain that could not learn in the way that brains usually learn'. It might be explained that someone 'could not keep children safe', perhaps that they 'could not see clearly' so that when they looked at 'their gorgeous baby girl' they did not see 'the beauty and goodness that everyone else knew was there'. Mental illness can be described as a 'kind of illness that makes people do strange things'. If there has been a bereavement by suicide the method might be described by saying that the person 'died because they took too many tablets' or that 'the rope was too tight on their neck', or 'a bullet went into their body'. It is not necessary to over explain. When the child is ready for more information they will ask. Keep the context for telling the story in mind when deciding how much detail to give.

Addressing cognitive distortions

The story also presents opportunities to address cognitive distortions and may contribute to the child, and the parent, re-evaluating any mistaken beliefs that they hold: 'and Johnny thought it was his job to keep his little sister safe. He didn't understand yet, because he was only (insert appropriate number) years old, that children are not in charge of what grownups do. Small boys can't stop big people from doing something that they have already decided to do.'

Reframing the child's actions

Children often give themselves a hard time and believe that they were 'weak' because they were not able to do something different during difficult experiences. We have an opportunity to reframe the child's coping strategy as being a strength: 'and Johnny's body knew exactly the right thing to do'. We can follow this by whatever he actually did (as long as you have reliable information in this regard) – for example, 'run away as fast as he could', or 'stay as still and as quiet as he possibly could' or 'just close his eyes and pretend to himself that the bad stuff wasn't happening again'.

Sequencing and integration

The touchstone story fosters integration and supports the child's future resiliency (Green, 2012) by bringing clarity to, and helping to make meaning of, confusing elements within their life story. It gives a coherent narrative and clear sequencing in relation to traumatic and/or disturbing events. Such stories need the containment of a beginning, middle and ending to make sense and allow the content to be successfully processed.

> Neurobiological evidence for traumatized children's affective and sensorimotor memory storage in the 'more primitive' somatic and visual areas of the brain has been presented by Van der Kolk (1996a). In the face of overwhelming experiences our facility for declaritative memory decreases and our ability to contextualise diminishes (Van der Kolk, 1996b). This results in a form of 'speechless terror' in which the limbic system is activated and Broca's area is deactivated (Van der Kolk 1996c), and we are unable to give narrative to our immediate experiences. Instead we are left with a more primitive sensory and somatic level of processing that does not facilitate us in being able to coherently understand and transfer the experience to long term memory.
>
> (Prendiville, 2014: 94)

Trauma also interferes with the ability to sequence. Children and adults who have been traumatized find it difficult to tell their story in an organized fashion. The play of traumatized children is similarly disorganized and accompanied by disruptions (Erikson, 1950; Chazan, 2002; Yasenik and Gardner, 2012). Gantt and Tinnin (2009) suggest that 'posttraumatic disorders involve nonverbal mental activity that escapes or overrides verbal thinking' (p. 148), and propose a protocol that 'aims to restore a sense of temporal order by developing a (visual) coherent narrative, re-contextualize fragmentation, associate non-verbal memories with verbal description and facilitate transfer of memories to past memory' (Prendiville, 2014: 89). When we present the child's story to them as part of our intake procedures we allow them to hear it, perhaps for the first time, as a coherent, properly sequenced narrative.

Making links between life events and presenting issues

A further aim or outcome of telling the story is that it may assist the family in making links between life events and presenting issues. In my experience it is quite common for parents not to see the connection between life events and emotional or behavioural difficulties. The story can help here: 'and after that Sally started to have trouble sleeping, eating and playing with her friends. She started to get pains in her tummy and often did not want Mummy to go out of her sight. She didn't even want to go to school anymore.'

Orientation to play therapy and the therapist's values

The touchstone story gives the therapist an opportunity to introduce themselves, and their job, in more detail so as to further help in reassuring the child and in structuring their relationship. It is also useful to present their own world-view in a way that might help the child understand how the therapist views their experiences. For example, the therapist who explains about the 'rules of the world' as described above is communicating the value they place on children being kept safe. Part of the story might say something like 'and then a wrong thing happened and the little girl got hurt. Oh, oh, that is not supposed to happen, (the offender) broke the rules!' There can also be a direct statement in the story: 'It is not OK for anyone to hurt boys and girls.' A commitment to safety comes in again at the end of the story when the therapist refers to the rules of the playroom: 'I told Mummy that I have one big rule in my playroom, and that is the safe rule. That means that I don't hurt children and children don't hurt me, and I am in charge of that.' This indicates that adults cannot delegate responsibility for safety to the child. Confidentiality can also be explained in the story and can include a reference to breaching confidentiality should child protection concerns arise: '(Therapist's name) will keep what happens in the playroom private except if she is worried about somebody not being safe or being hurt.'

Touchstone story structure for children with complex histories

So, we are getting a sense of the content of this more complex story and how is it structured. We will now look at the guidelines to refer to when preparing a story for a child with a complex history; there are obviously more stages involved than in our earlier example.

Complex history

1. Give the story a title.
2. The beginning of the story is set at a stage before any traumatic events occurred.
3. Emphasize the presence of any secure attachments or supportive adults and do not ignore positive life experiences.
4. Describe the difficult life event/s in child friendly language.
5. If grooming was involved include this.
6. Emphasize the child's coping.
7. Include psycho-educational component if appropriate, especially addressing cognitive distortions.
8. It may be appropriate to incorporate some elements of trauma debriefing into the story (for example, sensory elements, emotional context, fears).
9. Refer to any difficulties that ensued (including presenting problems).
10. Address any feelings of guilt or shame (normalizing and reframing).

> 11. Refer to parental responses and address any deficiencies.
> 12. Refer to the current presence of a supportive ally.
> 13. Include the referral, intake sessions and information that was made available to you.
> 14. Include references to the child's strengths and attractive qualities.
> 15. The story ends in the present tense – with the child attending the appointment and their story being told.

The first three points are the same as in the previous guidelines. However, in describing the complex events the writer needs to pay particular attention to ensuring that the language chosen will enable the child to attend to the story while remaining regulated. If grooming was involved, this will be described so that the family and the child begin to get an age-appropriate understanding of how they were manipulated. An emphasis on the child's coping, and reframing this as described earlier, if needed, can help the child remain calm. Attention is paid to ensuring that whenever content that might be distressing to the child is included, it is followed by content that will facilitate regulation. Psycho-educational content may be included, especially if the information acquired during the intake suggested that the child or family are holding mistaken beliefs in relation to dynamics, causes or consequences of the events.

It may be appropriate to incorporate some elements of trauma debriefing into the story. This can be particularly useful for children who have intrusive recollections that suggest that they have very fragmented memories. In these cases, I might refer to sensory elements (for example, a loud noise, flashing lights, a strong smell), or apparent emotions (for example, feeling very scared, worried or sad), or, occasionally, when the particular circumstances suggest it, refer to the child being so frightened that they thought they might die. After including the traumatic events, the story continues as in previous examples by addressing the emotional and behavioural difficulties, including the presenting problems.

The touchstone story can assist the adults in the child's life in understanding more clearly the dynamics of the child's experiences. Occasionally, parts of the story are included especially for the parents, particularly if they are holding inappropriate feelings of guilt or shame that interfere with the family's recovery. Because these feelings can be very difficult to overcome, the story will attempt to normalize (Graham and Reynolds, 2013) and reframe (Petriwskyj, 2013) these feelings in a way that will facilitate the family in moving on.

Telling the touchstone story using props

Ideally the story is told during the first session in the presence of the supportive ally. I do not use the playroom for this. I prefer to use the room in which I meet parents so that the child and I can leave and go to the playroom when the story is complete. Therapists who have the luxury of meeting the child during a home visit prior to starting therapy could tell the story during that visit and they can leave some photographs of themselves and the playroom and materials with the child. However, there have been times when the therapist has not been able to do either of these and they decide to introduce it later in the process. This has been useful for helping therapy that has become 'stuck' to move forward.

The therapist will choose props including characters and representations of important elements in the story (for example, an ambulance for a child taken to hospital following an accident). Choose neutral characters – avoid using Cruella De Vil for the new stepmother or a boxer for the parent who perpetrated domestic violence! In some cases, especially if there are not too many characters needed, it can be good to present a selection of small figures and invite the child to choose characters to represent each person needed, or even just to choose the character that represents themselves. Other options are to use puppets or art techniques for telling the story. Possibilities include drawing a time line, a river, or simply dividing a page into a number of sections to depict various scenes in the story. With older children, some therapists prefer to just read the story but this eliminates some of the psychological distancing that can be gained by having an external object to focus on. In general, it is best to use projective, small world, play when telling the story; projective play is a very effective medium for helping children process issues that are confusing to them and that interfere with their healthy emotional development.

One of the main benefits of using props when telling the story is that references to the difficult sections are projected onto the miniature characters, enabling the child to stay focused on the play scene. References to coping, support and safety may be addressed directly to the child and family as considered appropriate. The dramatic distance afforded by the use of miniature characters combined with the therapist's air of playfulness, enables the child to go on the journey with the central character – thus reducing stress and anxiety.

Some children will join in as the story is being told and it is fine to incorporate their input. When telling Tom, whose dog died suddenly, and his family the story, Tom interjected to say, 'He used to chase after the ball when I threw it for him.' The therapist might respond by saying, 'Yes, and I know he used to get so excited when you came home from school and you used to play together. You had so much fun together and you really miss him every day.' However, if the child ignores you continue with the story and focus most of your attention on the characters rather than the child. If the child resists, acknowledge this, and then focus your attention and direct the story towards the child's parent/s – 'to be sure I understood everything'.

As described earlier, it is important to use the correct name when referring to the toy used to represent the child. However, there are times, perhaps when referring to strengths, coping, or positive characteristics, when it is appropriate to say 'you' instead. When doing this it is a good idea to make eye contact with the child.

Reflecting on the use of the therapeutic touchstone technique

My personal experience has been that the therapeutic touchstone has a dramatic impact on the therapy process. I believe it reduces the child's involvement in limit testing, enables them to introduce personally relevant play (Norton and Norton, 2006, 2008) very early in the therapy process, and makes it safe for them to spontaneously disclose experiences that have previously been kept secret.

While this technique is directive in nature, it provides a foundation for play therapy that may subsequently be either non-directive or directive. My belief is that it supports the child in making use of the therapy space and therapeutic relationship more fully and more quickly than might otherwise be possible. I believe that Maslow's hierarchy of needs model sheds light on why this might be so.

For the purposes of this exploration I am going to focus on the five levels of need that Maslow initially identified: physiological, safety, love, esteem and self-actualization.

Maslow proposed that the first four levels of need are based on a deficiency model; we strive to fill the need for them when they are absent so as to restore or achieve a state of homeostasis. These four levels, from the most basic upwards, are associated with physiological needs, safety needs, the need to belong and be loved, and the need to feel good about ourselves. Only the fifth level is associated with striving for a more complete way of being, our motivation to fulfil our potential and self-actualize.

I suggest that humanistic play therapists could enhance their practice by paying attention to these five motivating factors and organismic needs when assessing information in relation to the child's world outside therapy (their lived world) and also when planning their play therapy services. In fact, I suggest that most already do so but may not use this framework to conceptualize it. I further contend that our assessment in relation to ensuring

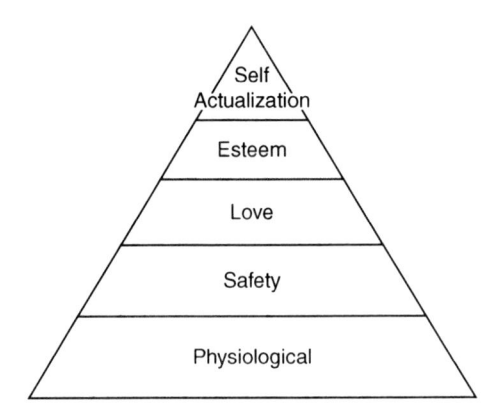

Figure 1.1 Maslow's hierarchy of needs diagram

that appropriate conditions exist in the child's lived world to make it safe enough for us to accept a referral, or to plan for any family based interventions that might be needed prior to accepting the referral, might focus first and foremost on whether the child's basic physiological needs, and their needs for safety and security, are currently being met. These seem to me to be essential if the child is to gain the maximum benefit from the therapy intervention. The higher level needs, for love and belonging, self-esteem, and self-actualization, can more easily be met during the therapy process if the therapist pays attention to both the therapy world and the lived world of their child client. I believe that these needs are linked to the quality of therapeutic interactions rather than the quantifiable elements that are intrinsic to the needs to feel safe, secure and having sufficient food, drinks, shelter, heat, and appropriate touch that are part and parcel of the first two levels.

In relation to providing play therapy, we should consider the levels of need in the provision of an appropriate supportive environment. We think of basic physiological needs when we schedule sessions (timing, provision of a warm room, access to bathroom). We consider safety needs when we equip our therapy room (safe materials, developmentally appropriate), and structure our interventions (structuring responses, limit setting). The humanistic therapist's commitment to the Rogerian core principles of unconditional positive regard, empathy and congruence, link in directly with the child's needs for acceptance and a sense of belonging. We embody these principles when we pay full attention to the child and when we accept them fully. When we recognize their efforts and achievements, highlight their ability to make choices and reflect back our experience of the child, we contribute to building their self-esteem, bringing us through the first four levels of Maslow's pyramid. The final level, the self-driven motivation towards self-actualization, is activated when these first four levels are not in deficiency mode. This is the heart and soul of therapy – enabling the client to become more authentic, fulfilled, spontaneous, self-reliant and emotionally healthy. If we truly believe that individuals have an inner drive that favours health over ill-health, maturity over stagnation and emotional well-being over maladjustment, then as therapists we are required to assist clients in activating this potential by providing the appropriate environment and conditions to alleviate deficiencies and enable their motivation towards this higher level of being. This might include removing any barriers within our therapy rooms and relationships and countering any blocks in the child's ability to benefit from circumstances that enrich their environments. We all know of children who are unable to benefit from favourable circumstances – for example, the child removed from an abusive home and placed with loving foster carers who cannot seem to fully experience the safety and acceptance that is now afforded to them. Or the child who is supported in educational and social settings but whose level of self-esteem remains low. Perhaps we can find clues as to the reasons for this by considering Maslow's hierarchy of needs?

The need to feel safe

The level that many children seem to be unable to integrate is that of experiencing the world as a safe place, even when dangers have been addressed and safety established. Perhaps this is because the child continues to test this safety and has never truly been convinced that it exists, that it is deliberate, or that it will last. Furthermore, perhaps one way of providing the richest ground for successful therapy (and facilitating the child to benefit from the core conditions offered in humanistic approaches to therapy) is to ensure as far as possible that the therapy context addresses this second level of need – the need for safety, security and freedom from fear – as fully and as early as possible. Without this, clients will not benefit fully from the acceptance and attention offered by the therapist as they will remain focused on the perceived deficiencies and therefore unable to experience love and a sense of belonging.

Green (2012) states that 'The number one factor in resiliency is feeling safe in one's environment' (p.13) and highlights the importance of safety in developing supportive relationships. The touchstone story is designed to contribute to meeting the child's needs for safety and security by countering some of the confusion they may feel and thus making it easier to address unresolved issues. I believe that this enables children to make better use of the acceptance and recognition that we offer in therapy – thereby increasing their potential to self- actualize. Further benefits are that we demonstrate to the child that we are including them as an equal, we are communicating in an open, honest and child friendly manner. This helps address the power imbalance that usually exists in adult/child relationships and can fast track the therapy process safely. This intervention can be used regardless of whether the therapist plans on working directively or non-directively. While it is a very focused and therapist chosen intervention, it only lasts six minutes and ideally is told before the child comes into the playroom for the first time. This frees up the therapist to allow the child to take the lead in play, if they wish to work this way. It brings the child's life story into the therapy in a child friendly way, allowing it to inform their symbolic play and story-making, and reduces the pressure on the therapist to engage directively. It recognizes the child as the expert on his or her own process. The therapist is then free to make clinical judgments in relation to interventions as personally relevant play (Norton and Norton, 2006, 2008) emerges and play disruptions and/or repetitive themes emerge.

It is very common for the child to ask for the story again at a later stage. It can be repeated in the same way as for the first telling, or the child may wish to contribute actively to the content or story-telling process. Some children wish to add in more detail in the re-telling. Some children like to have a hard copy of the story and may add drawings to depict some of the content or the characters involved.

Conclusion

While I have described the therapeutic touchstone in the way that I use it, others may wish to adapt or change it to suit their own approach to working therapeutically with children and adolescents. The important point is to work to ensure that it is a positive experience for the child and their family and that it remains a playful experience that provides containment, offers relief and provides a solid foundation for therapy.

Key points

1. The therapeutic touchstone is a play-based intervention in which the therapist uses story and toys to present a synopsis of significant elements in the child's life story to the child and their carer.
2. A simple structure is used when the child is experiencing simple emotional or behavioural difficulties and/or issues related to difficulties in adjustment.

3. A more complex structure, incorporating psycho-educational content, is used when the child has a complex history and/or has experienced significant interpersonal trauma.
4. Maslow's hierarchy of needs model might assist us in understanding why this intervention could facilitate the child in feeling safe and foster development of the therapeutic relationship.

References

Chazan, S. E. (2002). *Profiles of play: Assessing and observing structure and process in play therapy*. London: Jessica Kingsley Publications.
Davis, N. (1985). *Therapeutic stories to heal abused children*. Oxon Hill, MD: Psychological Associates of Oxon Hill.
Erikson, E. H. (1950). *Childhood and society*. New York: Norton.
Gantt, L. and Tinnin, L. W. (2009). Support for a neurobiological view of trauma with implications for art therapy. *The Arts in Psychotherapy*, 36, 148–153.
Graham, P. and Reynolds, S. (2013). *Cognitive Behaviour Therapy for Children and Families*. Cambridge: CUP.
Green, E. (2012). Fostering resiliency in traumatized adolescents: Integrating play and evidenced-based interventions. *Playtherapy*, June, 10–14.
Hartman, C. R. and Burgess, A. W. (1988). Information processing of trauma: Case application of a model. *Journal of Interpersonal Violence*. 3 (4), 443–457.
Levy, A. J. (2008). The therapeutic action of play in the psychodynamic treatment of children: A critical analysis. *Clinical Social Work Journal*, 36, 281–291.
Norton, C. and Norton, B. E. (2006). Experiential play therapy. In C. E. Schaefer and H. G. Kaduson (eds), *Contemporary play therapy: Theory, research, and practice* (pp. 28–54). New York: Guilford Press.
Norton, C. and Norton, B. E. (2008). *Reaching children through play therapy: An experiential approach* (3rd edn). Denver, CO: White Apple Press.
Petriwskyj, A. (2013). Reflections on talk about natural disasters by early childhood educators and directors. *Australian Journal of Communication*, 40 (1), 87–102.
Prendiville, E. (2014). Abreaction. In C. E. Schaefer and A. A. Drewes (eds) *The Therapeutic Powers of Play: 20 Core Agents of Change* (2nd edn), pp. 83–102. Hoboken, NJ: Wiley & Sons.
Rogers, R. C. (1980). *A Way of Being*. New York: Houghton Mifflin Company.
Sunderland, M. (2000). *Using storytelling as a therapeutic tool with children*. London: Speechmark.
Van der Kolk, B. A. (1996a). The body keeps the score: Approaches to the psychobiology of posttraumatic stress disorder. In B. Van der Kolk, A. McFarlane and L. Weisaeth (eds), *Traumatic stress: The effects of*

overwhelming experience on mind, body and society (pp. 214–241). New York: Guilford Press.

Van der Kolk, B. A. (1996b). The complexity of adaptation to trauma: Self-regulation, stimulus discrimination, and characterological development. In B. Van der Kolk, A. McFarlane and L. Weisaeth (eds), *Traumatic stress: The effects of overwhelming experience on mind, body and society* (pp. 182–213). New York: Guilford Press.

Van der Kolk, B. A. (1996c). Trauma and memory. In B. Van der Kolk, A. McFarlane and L. Weisaeth (eds), *Traumatic stress: The effects of overwhelming experience on mind, body and society* (pp. 279–302). New York: Guilford Press.

Van der Kolk, B., McFarlane, A. and Weisaeth, L. (eds). (1996). *Traumatic stress: The effects of overwhelming experience on mind, body and society*. New York: Guilford Press.

Yasenik, L. and Gardner, K. (2012). *Play therapy dimensions model: A decision making guide for integrative play therapists*. Philadelphia, PA: Jessica Kingsley Publications.

2

The consciousness dimension in play therapy

Sharpening the play therapist's focus and skills

Lorri Yasenik and Ken Gardner

The case of Gina is used to study the emergence of consciousness during a series of play therapy sessions. This study exemplifies an increase in consciousness as related to increasing indices of self-awareness. We begin this clinical exploration by asking, 'Why should we be interested in consciousness at all?' Consciousness is related to degrees of self-knowledge and self-awareness and most, if not all, therapies are interested in self-development, self-agency, self-efficacy and self-awareness, even if the focus is not primarily on 'talk' as the main form of intervention. James' (1890) theory, which was re-embraced during postmodernism, is viewed once again as a current important construct (Harter, 2012). The I-self as knower, the Me-self as known, and the idea of multiple Me-selves as part of self-development, is used here to examine the emerging consciousness in sandplay therapy with a ten-year-old girl. Adult self-theories cannot be compared to the self-theories of the developing child based on numerous cognitive limitations. Harter notes:

> That is, the I-self, in its role of constructor of the Me-self does not, in childhood, possess the capacities to create a hierarchically organized system of postulates that are internally consistent, coherently organized, testable or empirically valid. In fact, it is not until *late adolescence* if not early adulthood that the abilities to construct such a self-portrait potentially emerge.
>
> (2012, p. 9)

Harter (2012) therefore argues for the analysis of the I-self at various stages of development, because the I-self impacts on the emergence of the

Me-self. The focus on developmental changes also allows the therapist to address levels of differentiation and integration (two levels of self-theory). Through differentiation, increasing cognitive abilities will help the child to differentiate experiences. Through integration, higher order generalizations can be made about the self as related to traits and abilities.

It is important for play therapists to have good observation skills in following and supporting the emergence of consciousness in play therapy. An awareness of the indications of rising consciousness in play highlights a child's emerging sense of self and self-awareness. The case of Gina exemplifies the client/therapist interaction as moments of consciousness become apparent. The Play Therapy Dimensions Model (Yasenik and Gardner, 2012) was referred to when working with Gina as it is a model of tracking the two main dimensions in play therapy: consciousness and directiveness.

An overview of the Play Therapy Dimensions Model

Recognizing that play therapists are increasingly moving toward integrative thinking, the Play Therapy Dimensions Model (Yasenik and Gardner, 2012) was developed as a decision-making model for the intentional, integrative play therapist.

One of the primary integrative approaches in the adult psychotherapy literature is referred to as Theoretical Integration (Wachtel, 1977). In this approach, the therapist's case conceptualization and interventions are based on an understanding of two or more theoretical frameworks. Authors concur that a common adult-based decision-making process would be valuable when taking an integrative approach (Beutler and Clarkin, 1990; Street *et al.* 2000). However, decision-making guidelines or structures are noticeably lacking for integrative psychotherapists (Schottenbauer *et al.* 2007). Play therapists would equally benefit from accessing decision-making parameters to optimize treatment planning and interventions. Going one step beyond this essential need, emphasis must be placed on active and intentional tracking of the play therapy process on a moment-to-moment, session-to-session basis, based on a decision-making framework. When approached from this perspective, the intentional, integrative play therapist actively examines the *who*, *what*, *when*, *why* and *how* of play therapy.

One theoretical approach to integrative decision-making, bounded rationality, takes note of the practical limitations for therapists such as resources, time and knowledge (Gigerenzer, 2001) and emphasizes the need to describe timely ways to gather information and make decisions. In short, this approach stresses the need to know *where* to focus and the parameters for determining *when* or *why* to use certain techniques or

The consciousness dimension in play therapy | 31

interventions. The Play Therapy Dimensions Model (Yasenik and Gardner, 2012) is consistent with an integrative conceptualization process, as it offers the play therapist decision-making structures for looking at the interaction of client-therapist-treatment factors. An examination of this interaction is accomplished by conceptualizing the play therapy process according to two primary dimensions: directiveness and consciousness.

As represented in Figure 2.1, the two primary dimensions intersect, forming four quadrants: Quadrant I – Active Utilization; Quadrant II – Open Discussion and Exploration; Quadrant III – Non-Intrusive Responding; and Quadrant IV – Co-facilitation. Each of the four quadrants is identified by the therapist's activities and the child's direction and level of consciousness during the play therapy session. Depending on the case conceptualization, and theoretical approaches taken by the play therapist, a therapist might choose to focus therapy activities primarily in one quadrant. Alternatively there may be a number of indicators that suggest movement is required amongst the four quadrants. Consistent with an integrative approach, there is no prescriptive order for movement between the quadrants. Furthermore, movement may occur within a session, across sessions, or as the therapy process evolves. As will be illustrated in the case of Gina, the conceptualization of the two primary domains, and the resulting four quadrants, assists the therapist in navigating the complex client-therapist-treatment interactions in order to tailor the treatment approach.

The directiveness dimension represents the therapist's activity with respect to the degree of immersion in the play. The term immersion refers to the degree to which the therapist enters and actively takes part in the

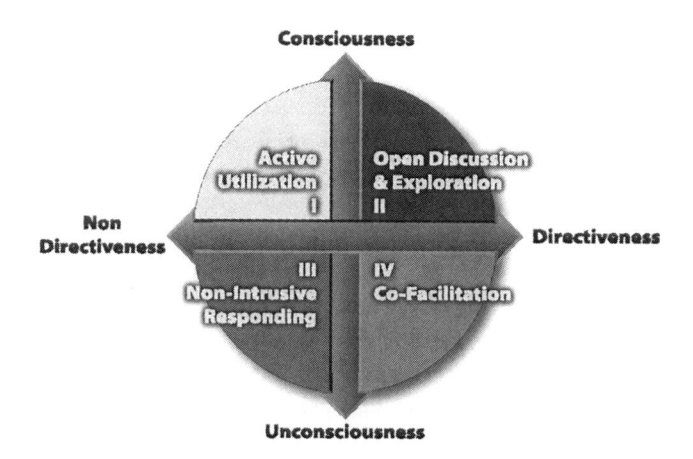

Figure 2.1 Play Therapy Dimensions diagram. Reproduced with permission from Yasenik and Gardner (2012, p. 34)

play. At the far left side of this dimension the therapist is tracking the play through observation and reflection and is not involved in interactive play with the child. At the far right side of this dimension, the therapist has entered the play as a co-facilitator and is actively taking part in elaborating and extending the play.

The directiveness dimension is perhaps the most familiar dimension to play therapists, regardless of their theoretical orientation. However, there is much debate amongst practitioners, often polarizing in nature, concerning preferences for working in a directive or non-directive manner (Yasenik and Gardner, 2012). The non-directive side of the directiveness continuum is most clearly evidenced in the child-centred approach to play therapy. However, close inspection of child-centred approaches suggests that variations exist in the way contemporary experts (Guerney, 2001; Landreth, 2002; Van Fleet *et al.* 2010; Wilson and Ryan, 2005) think about certain strategies and non-directive skills. Accordingly, as discussed by Yasenik and Gardner (2012), some non-directive/child-centred play therapists will be seen as moving back and forth along the directiveness dimension. Consistent with this understanding, the reader will notice, in the case discussion that follows, the therapist at times provides a story-stem direction that initially places this activity on the right side of this dimension. The therapist then returns the lead to the child and the child leads and directs the play, demonstrating movement back to the left side of the directiveness dimension.

The consciousness dimension reflects the child's representation of consciousness in play activities and verbalizations. For the integrative play therapist who seeks to understand the unique needs of each child and respond in an intentional manner, there is great value in knowing how to conceptualize movement along this dimension. For example, an understanding of child moderating factors, such as the nature and strength of the child's defences and the child's worldview, is critical when we are helping a child to reorganize or make sense of a disturbing experience (Yasenik and Gardner, 2012). This work may be accomplished at a lower level of the child's self-awareness – through the play metaphor – or at a higher level of awareness – through a process of interpretation or open discussion. Depending on the therapist's understanding of the child's defences and need for distance from the issue, the therapist might weave up and down this dimension, at times bringing issues into higher levels of conscious awareness through interpretations or restatements of affect. Alternatively, the therapist could remain working in the play metaphor and elaborate the play to assist in the child's drive to gain mastery and re-organize the experience. Through an examination of indicators of shifting levels of self-awareness and consciousness, the therapist working with Gina uses this information to gauge the child's readiness to incorporate information and affect at higher levels of consciousness, on a moment-to-moment, session-by-session basis. Note how the therapist observes that the child's play is at times accompanied by verbalizations (i.e. where the I-self reflects on the Me-self), indicating that the child is working with a certain level of conscious awareness. At other times, Gina uses play scenarios and objects in a less conscious and more symbolic or metaphorical manner, representing lower levels of self-awareness – probably because she needs distance and protection from troublesome thoughts or feelings.

The four quadrants provide an organizing structure for play therapists. No matter what theoretical orientation a therapist primarily draws from, he/she will be able to identify the levels of their directiveness, immersion and the degree to which they facilitate the child's conscious awareness of emerging play themes and activities. Rather than anchoring each quadrant name or title to a specific theoretical model or play therapy approach, the quadrant titles reflect elements of the client-therapist-treatment interactions, as conceptualized by the two primary dimensions – directiveness and consciousness. To illustrate this further, when working in Quadrant III, Non-Intrusive Responding, the therapist is less immersed in the play – the child leads the play and the therapist acts as a *non-intrusive* responder. On the far right hand side of the directiveness dimension, but occurring below the mid-point on the consciousness dimension, is Quadrant IV, Co-facilitation. When working in this quadrant, the play therapist enters the play, either at the invitation of the child or because the therapist has observed a number of themes or patterns, and makes a decision to test a hypothesis or elaborate the play by inserting comments, actions or soft interpretations in the context of the play. This role would seem familiar to those working from an Adlerian approach, where emphasis is placed on an egalitarian relationship in which there is a sense of shared power and responsibility (Kottman, 2003). To maintain this relationship, the therapist may enter and elaborate the play after tracking a number of patterns and themes in the child's play. The degree of therapist immersion increases considerably in Quadrant IV compared to Quadrant III. This signifies that the therapist's role shifts from a non-intrusive responder to that of a co-facilitator.

Active Utilization is identified in the upper left corner of Figure 2.1, Quadrant 1. In this quadrant the child initiates the play using his/her own metaphors or verbalizations. This quadrant is placed on the non-directive side of the diagram and is differentiated from Quadrant III (which is also on the left side of the diagram) due to the intermittent interpretive comments initiated by the therapist that may trigger conscious responses from the child. Simply stated, during the play process, therapists sometimes expand the play metaphor, through making reflective/interpretive comments, thereby expanding the play into higher levels of conscious awareness. Typically, active utilization is entered into in a brief, time-sensitive way. This quadrant will be familiar to therapists who believe in using interpretive comments to help children reorganize dissociated affect or to work through material in a more conscious manner.

Quadrant II, Open Discussion and Exploration, is located in the upper right corner of Figure 2.1. A therapist working in this quadrant would be observed as initiating and structuring play activities relative to the child's presenting problem – such as anxiety, depression, or poor self-control. When working in this quadrant, the therapist will often introduce the child to concrete, highly conscious interventions. Additionally, the therapist is viewed as primarily using a developmentally sensitive, cognitive play therapy approach, in which he/she engages in open discussions and conscious processing of the child's presenting issues. Quadrant II is considered to be the place where therapists are observed introducing the highest degree of consciousness and directiveness to the child.

The Play Therapy Dimensions Model assists therapists to consider movement from their original point of intervention or approach to other intervention possibilities. It must be emphasized that the model is not prescriptive and does not presume that movement has to occur. Rather, the model invites the therapist to view the play therapy process on a moment-to-moment basis and see therapeutic activities as dynamic, based on a number of factors such as the stage of the therapeutic process, the responses of the child to the therapist, the child's play skills and the child's drive and direction in therapy.

Understanding the dimension of consciousness

Surprisingly, despite the long history of the scientific study of consciousness, as well as the fact that the field of psychology initially began as a science of consciousness well over one hundred years ago (Chalmers, 2005), the impact and importance of this dimension seems to have escaped our conscious minds as play therapists (Yasenik and Gardner, 2012). Yet, on the most core or basic level, consciousness is viewed as a critical biological function that allows us to know emotions, such that when consciousness is impaired, so are emotions (Damasio, 1999).

Historically, the dynamic psychiatry systems espoused by Janet, Freud, Adler and Jung preferred a dual concept/model of the mind – a conscious and unconscious ego. Depth psychology claimed to have a way to explore the unconscious mind, such as Freud's idea of analysing resistance and transference. Others, such as Jung, were part of the 'unmasking' trend, and were involved in an examination of unconscious motivations (Ellenberger, 1970).

As noted by O'Connor and Braverman (2009), we now have a neurological understanding of the basic emotional operating system of the mammalian brain, as well as of the conscious and unconscious states which they generate. In examining the characteristics of play O'Connor (2000) hypothesizes that there is a 'flow', or a centring of attention. The implication for the play therapist is that we should be concerned about *how*, *when* and *why* we focus or centre the child's attention during play activities. In other words, the play therapist should act in an intentional and thoughtful manner.

Damasio (1999) asserts that there are different levels of consciousness. The most primary level, referred to as core consciousness, provides us with a sense of self in the here-and-now. On the other hand, the complex or extended type of consciousness provides us with a more elaborate sense of self, offering up an identity or personhood that includes past and anticipated future experiences. As discussed by Damasio, 'Extended consciousness still hinges on the same core "you", but that "you" is now connected to the lived past and the anticipated future that are part of your autobiographical record.' (1999, p. 196). Damasio relates these two levels of consciousness to the two kinds of self – the core self and the autobiographical self. Damasio indicates that the human mind is constantly being split between the part that stands for the *known* and the part that stands for the *knower*. He further postulates that there is a 'proto-self',which is a temporary neural pattern that represents our state, moment-to-moment. As such, the proto-self participates in the process of knowing, versus being a storehouse of knowledge. From this standpoint, consciousness is the part of the mind concerned with the apparent sense of self and knowing; consciousness must be present if feelings are to influence the person beyond the immediate here-and-now. As Damasio asserts, there is a significant difference between having a 'feeling' and 'knowing that we have a feeling' (1999, p. 32).

In Damasio's model, the core self does not interpret anything. The proposed underlying neuroanatomical structures are seen to simply form an imaged, non-verbal, second-order account of how the organism is affected by the processing of an object. As discussed by Damasio (1999), by the end of the nineteenth century, in his exploration of emotions and the mind, William James offered a similar accounting of this process and, in spite of its incompleteness in terms of brain anatomy, developed a model that provides a cornerstone for our current conceptualization of consciousness. Damasio states, 'Just as William James would have wished, nearly the whole brain is engaged in a conscious state' (1999, p. 194).

Over the last century we have had several shifts in how we think about the self, moving from the romanticism period, through to modernism and postmodernism (Harter, 2012). In taking a contemporary, postmodern approach to self-development, one that examines cognitive-developmental as well as sociocultural influences, Harter (2012) argues that James' (1890) distinction between the I-self as the actor or knower and the Me-self as the object of one's knowledge has proven viable over the decades and is a recurrent construct in many theoretical treatments of the self. In fact, James (1890) stated that the individual creates multiple Me-selves, paralleling the different types of social roles one performs over the course of life. As discussed by Harter (2012), James postulated that the conscious conflict of the different 'Me's' arose because of the incompatibility of the various social roles that the individual must negotiate. Harter (2012) further emphasizes that James has come back into favour with cognitive theories of self because it is readily agreed that people naturally look at themselves as objects of self-reflection.

Taking James' theories into the developmental laboratory, so to speak, Harter (2012) has examined how the I-self in each developmental stage directly impacts the Me-self, namely the self-theory being constructed. Further, Harter (2012) posits that there are sub-stages in the progression of self-understanding, and that these levels build on and transform one another. Essentially, there is a process of differentiation and integration that is part of the development of our self-theory.

> With regard to differentiation, emerging cognitive abilities allow the individual to create self-evaluations that differ across various domains of experience. Moreover, they permit the older child to distinguish between real and ideal self-concepts, which can then be compared to one another, creating discrepancies that have further consequences for the self.
> (Harter, 2012, p. 10)

The process of integration implies that as cognitive abilities arise over the course of development, the child can construct higher-order generalizations about the self in the form of trait labels – such as thinking of oneself as athletic or smart. Particularly relevant to the case of Gina is that during middle childhood abilities emerge which permit the child to construct a concept of his/her worth as a person, namely an evaluation of their global self-esteem (Harter, 2012).

We would be remiss to refer to this dimension without emphasizing that when working with young children, their capacity for conscious 'awareness' must be considered from a developmental perspective. Interested play therapists may wish to review Zelazo's (2004) Levels of Consciousness model, which adopts a developmental perspective and examines how five degrees of consciousness gradually emerge in infants and children. This model is based on the assumption that there is a mechanism of recursion, which takes place at each level, whereby the contents of consciousness are fed back into consciousness so that they become accessible to consciousness at a higher level. It is assumed that with each higher level of consciousness, the child's mental experiences become qualitatively richer and easier to recall. As a result, the child's conscious control of behaviour increases.

Finally, our understanding of the consciousness dimension can be furthered by discussing Siegel's (1999) work on mindsight, and his emphasis on the development of Me and You maps. Briefly, Siegel asserts that mindsight is the ability to look within and perceive the mind. In part, mindsight develops as a result of integrative processes such as the attuned adult reflecting back to the child their sense of the child's experiences and thoughts. Siegel (1999) argues that to develop mindsight one must reduce levels of reactivity and increase the ability to attend. Essentially, there is the need to recruit higher areas of the brain to override stress signals from the brainstem and limbic areas. As highlighted in the case of Gina, the therapist carefully titrated sandplay experiences to assist in this child's ability to attend to certain emotional states. In this manner, the therapeutic process gradually shifted the child's conscious focus of attention. Consistent with Siegel's model (1999), the therapist worked to increase internal and external communication, which in itself requires openness and awareness to perceive the self.

Siegel (1999) emphasizes that in order to increase mindsight the therapeutic process needs to provide a means of integration. Harter (2012), working from a cognitive, developmental framework, also emphasizes that at each stage of development children must work through a process of differentiation and integration. Let us now turn to the case of Gina to examine how the play therapy process unfolded, helping this child gain a stronger, more integrated, sense of self.

Case study – Gina

Ten-year-old Gina was referred for counselling by her parents in collaboration with the family doctor. During the parent intake session, Gina was described as a somewhat anxious child who had developed an overwhelming fear of 'throwing up'. The onset of Gina's fear (which had now turned to phobic proportions) had occurred two years previously when she had gotten violently ill and threw up every ten minutes for an entire evening. This event was described as extreme and quite sudden. Generally, Gina did not often get sick and this would have been her first experience of extreme illness. Reportedly, Gina was an above average student with good friends. She came from a very supportive, healthy, functioning home with highly sensitive and caring parents.

Gina's parents noted no body image issues, and no significant anxiety about anything else. She did not historically worry a lot, but was now extremely worried any time there may be a possibility of herself, her sibling, family members or friends throwing up or needing to throw up. This also extended to anyone close to her having any minor symptoms of illness. Once aware of anyone feeling symptoms of minor sickness, Gina would complain of having severe stomach aches. Her parents took Gina to the doctor to rule out stomach issues, reflux problems and celiac disease. Gina generally eats very well; however, she began to get nervous around meal times and would go to the bathroom during meals 'in case' she had to throw up. Gina's worry and concern about throwing up occurred each bedtime at home (although she went on many sleep-overs with no concern). She would report a stomach ache to her parents and lay awake for hours, crying. If her sibling or a family member noted he/she had a headache during the day or a stomach ache or that he/she simply did not feel well, this information could set Gina into tears, and she would rock herself at night in a foetal position noting she was scared and worried for the 'sick' person.

Gina's parents tried all of the logical behavioural and emotional interventions including lying with her at night and providing her with soothing messages, providing music for her to listen to, doing yoga with her before bed and, as more of a placebo effect, giving her some over the counter drugs for reflux and stomach issues at bedtime. Gina had begun to associate various events together (a kind of magical thinking) as a way to explain her reactions. For instance, she thought that a visit from her grandfather, which had corresponded with her getting sick once, would cause her to be sick again. She associated pizza, curry, and liquorice with getting sick also as these were foods she associated with a day she had been sick (after the major throwing-up incident). Gina asked her mother if she could 'get some help' to get rid of her problem.

Where to begin?

I (Lorri Yasenik) briefly began to work with Gina in Quadrant II, Open Discussion and Exploration, by asking her about her concerns from her point of view and then by giving her an instruction related to her self-described feeling states. Once given some direction, Gina then moved to non-directive work in Quadrant III, Non-Intrusive Responding. I primarily stayed working with the metaphors provided by Gina and my play-based actions could be observed as weaving between Quadrant III, Non-Intrusive Responding and Quadrant IV, Co-facilitation. By continuing to work within the metaphor, Gina could symbolize her thoughts and feelings and she could have an externalization experience of her fear state. The affective and interpersonal processes of the play-based sessions could potentially lead Gina to experience increased adaptive abilities such as creative thinking, problem-solving and new social behaviour.

Session one: The scared girl and cat

Gina was a highly verbal child who appeared eager to talk about her 'problem'. Her goal was 'I want to get rid of the feeling'. Knowing that sickness is a physiological feeling, I also asked her about what emotions she felt when her problem came up. She noted, 'I'm afraid, but I am also very sad. When I feel these two things I get upset and I get a stomach ache.' I asked Gina what things she had already tried to help make her feel better. Gina said she sometimes wrote in her journal, watched an imaginary 'show' in her head or drew to make herself feel 'distracted'. Although Gina was quite verbal and could have 'talked' about her problem, this had already been tried with her parents, the family doctor and her grandparents. I realized that if Gina were to shift her feeling state and gain control over her situation, she would need to approach the problem from a less direct and less conscious way.

Verbally rationalizing her situation with Gina had not helped her. Siegel points out, 'Emotions are primarily non-conscious mental processes. In their essence, they create a state of readiness for action, for "motion", disposing us to behave in particular ways in the environment' (1999, p. 132). From the neuropsychology perspective, the amygdala (an appraisal centre of the brain) provides a complex feedback process without the requirement of consciousness. The amygdala may have responded to Gina's initial severe vomiting experience by sending signals to any similar or earlier representations of the visual processing system, thereby producing an attentional and perceptual representation that registered the severe vomiting experience as dangerous.

Siegel (1999) uses fear of a dog as an example and refers to the amygdala registering the visual input of a dog as dangerous which establishes an appraisal-arousal process that creates a fear state and then sends this feedback back to the visual system. This brain-activated process thereby sets up a future perceptual bias towards fear of dogs. In Gina's case, one hypothesis was that she had registered vomiting as 'dangerous'. Any incoming stimulus that was similar appeared to be setting off danger signals that led her to experience a fear state that was not easily mediated by verbal discussion. The non-conscious wiring of the brain is a rapid process. My discussions with Gina's parents indicated that she had been experiencing hyper-arousal for a couple of years by the time I began to see her, which meant that her ongoing perceptions of any minor sickness activated her arousal system leading her to respond as if she would become 'out of control sick' again. A learned feedback loop appeared to have been established. Studies of anxiety disorders and phobias have been linked to this neurobiological explanation (Siegel, 1999).

I asked Gina if she would go to the sandtray and choose miniatures that reminded her of the 'scared' and 'sad' feelings and place them in the tray. She struggled to begin and asked me to choose what those characters would be and noted, 'I don't know, what do you mean?' I did not step in to help her choose, rather I just asked her about what she thought the sad/scared feelings might look like. Gina looked carefully and chose a very tiny girl figure that in her words 'looked scared enough' and a small cat and placed them together in the sand. I then used an externalizing construct and asked her to choose an object that could be the 'trickster', the one that tricks her into thinking she will throw up. She chose a dark character with slanted eyes standing on top of something – making the character tall. Gina placed this character on the other side of the tray. She then chose a bridge structure to be in the middle and placed a lion ('not a big lion,' she said) peering out at the trickster character from an opening in the bridge on the same side as the tiny girl and cat figures. Before she left the session I gave Gina a new journal and the pictures of her scene. I asked her to come up with some statements that the girl and cat could say to the trickster. Gina eagerly agreed.

Understanding the play process: working with increasing consciousness with Gina

Although there is no single way practitioners view working with consciousness, Siegel has raised the idea of the working memory as one way of understanding conscious awareness. The lateral prefrontal cortex is the area of the brain that takes perceptual representations (external sources and internal sources from imagination) and functionally connects these representations. The lateral prefrontal cortex region of the brain modulates attention, creating an attentional spotlight (Baddeley, 1992). There is a view that the idea of 'consciousness' makes continuous a set of discontinuous representations of sights, sounds, thoughts, bodily states, and self-reflections (Dennett, 1991; Siegel, 1999). The theory is that working memory can only focus on small amounts of information at a time, ordered in a linear or serial fashion. Therefore, finding a way to work with Gina that did not overwhelm her or increase her distress was my goal. Using the sandtray as a means of creating an attentional 'spotlight' for Gina's exploration of her self appeared appropriate. The once discontinuous experience that Gina had around her sudden and severe illness (fragmented representations) may be made more continuous through working with symbols in a play-based way.

The first action taken by me was to direct Gina's attention to externalized objects that could symbolize some of her previous discontinuous representations. Gina carefully chose items she could relate to. She was seemingly unaware that these items could represent parts of her experience of her fear of throwing up. The I-self eventually becomes conscious of the Me-self through what Harter (2012) refers to as an object of reflection and evaluation. For Gina, the I-self (the knower) was busy choosing things for the sandtray. The Me-self was not yet known in relation to these representative objects. They were simply items in a tray that I directed her to begin to have a relationship with through writing in her journal. A type of internal dialoguing began.

Session two: 'Added protection'

Gina brought her journal back to the next session. She quickly noted she had written some things down, but said they were 'not any good.' She was not sure if it was what I had wanted. She read her statements and said they were not very powerful. I asked her if she could go to the sandtray again and find the scared girl, cat, trickster and the lion. She found them all and again noted, 'the lion is still small'. I then asked if she could find a helper for the lion. Again, like last session, Gina said she did not know what I meant and was not immediately able to choose anything. I asked her about what could be helpful to the lion. I did not step in to assist her in choosing characters. I noticed Gina's deference to me for direction and approval.

Gina found a gorilla for the lion, she added a tiger and some more barriers between the girl and cat and the trickster. She stated, 'we need something for the little ones'. She found a hut to put over the girl and cat. She placed a wizard near the scared girl and cat's house. Of importance, Gina uses the I-self and notes, 'I think I need more protection and magic'. I printed the pictures taken of the sand scene and asked Gina, as homework, to write messages all the way around the pictures from the gorilla and the lion to the trickster as well as from the wizard to the trickster. The idea of magic was intriguing. The direction to engage in internal dialoguing with the externalized objects continued.

Session three: 'The Wizard's World'

Gina said at the beginning of session three that she did not know why, but she got more stomach aches during weekdays than on weekends. During this session, the I-self illuminated the need for more personal power and protection. This child was highly protected by family, and the idea of her need for an increased internal sense of personal power was observed. Was Gina searching for inner power so she could gain a sense of mastery over her fear?

During session three, I followed Gina's previous I-self direction regarding her earlier reference to the wizard and power and asked her to create 'The Wizard's World'. This world was constructed on one half of the sand tray with a line drawn down the middle. The wizard's side of the world had a wizard and a king (as his friend) and there were a few other mythical characters that lived near the wizard, such as dwarfs, magical swords, two fairy sisters, a unicorn, a glass elephant and a fish. The king and wizard were 'hidden' by a blue piece of fabric (water). They could see out, but no one could see in. There was a carefully hidden, large power stone in the wizard's side with many things around it to protect it – trees, swords etc. Gina said, 'No one has found this one; so hopefully the wizard will find this one and help me.' Here the I-self is bringing forward information for the Me-self during the play session. All focus is still on the items, but the I-self attempts to reveal needs to the Me-self.

On the other side, Gina created a mythical forest where the bad animals lived and six power stones were buried. The wizard's side made a clear path to this 'dark' side and at night the characters on the wizard's side sleep and in the day they go to the mythical forest looking for more power stones. Gina noted, 'They work all day to find a stone.' Gina further stated, 'The characters in the wizard's world come out to help the girl and cat (scared and sad parts of self) *when the trickster comes to threaten them.' According to Gina, the trickster takes a break during weekends and daytime as she does not get stomach aches or worry about throwing up during these times. At the end of this session, I asked Gina to choose a power stone to take home and use at night. Gina was pleased and noted, 'This will be a surprise for the trickster.'* The I-self was beginning to increase the likelihood of the Me-self consciously knowing more about the fear state. Small bits of information were being illuminated so that Gina could consciously know what was happening for her and how to self-manage the phobic responses.

Session four: The cat and girl's world – a turning point

Gina reported she had taken the power stone to a sleepover and that although she had been worried, the stone apparently helped and she did not have a stomach ache that night. I decided to assist Gina in further illuminating the fear and sadness states as during the last session she had put forth needing to know she could access more personal power. I asked Gina to create the cat and girl's world in the sandtray. Gina stated, 'I think they have been living in such a safe and protected world, they were not used to unsafe and scary things happening.' This was yet another indication of the emergence of consciousness for Gina. The I-self appeared to be illuminating a level of awareness that the Me-self needed to know. I could have simply said this to Gina during therapy, as I had come to understand how important and special she was to her parents, but that would not have been helpful. She was the youngest child, whom her parents protected and cherished. The overprotection appeared to slow down the development of self in areas of self-efficacy, self-competence and self-confidence.

For this sand scene, Gina used a tiger that was, in her words, a kind helper. She also put in many other kind and caring figures. The tiger helper only came out at night. She further stated, 'The tiger is used to the idea that bad things can happen – yeah and you can survive it.' This appeared to me to be another level of consciousness emerging. The trickster apparently did not know this world existed and, according to Gina, the trickster does not go after people who are not that scared or ones who are stronger. She noted the roles of a number of helpers in the scene and said again that this place was not a place for the 'weak', but it was a place for nice people. Again there were jewels and stones of value and the centre of the scene was made of valuable jewels, trees and flowers. When asked later if the girl and cat come out of their house at night and could they ask the tiger for help, Gina's answer indicated higher levels of consciousness as she did not stay in the metaphor, but rather stated, 'I was ok last night. . .well my stomach hurt for a little while. Tonight I think I will have a stomach ache though because tomorrow I have to have a vaccine at school.' Gina quickly returned to the metaphor and said that 'the trickster was counting on the girl and cat being weak – but really they just needed to get stronger.' My goal here was to further facilitate connection with Gina's inner strength. In her scene were two figures she called royalty who were consultants to her in the girl and cat's world. I asked her to obtain some messages from the royalty to the cat and girl about 'being stronger than they think' and Gina's answer was, 'They also need to learn that bad things happen, but you survive'.

Session five: Gaining power

Gina arrived at her session and told me that she had come home from school last week and thrown up. She calmly called her mother to tell her and she said she was not scared and did not have a big reaction, nor did she have a stomach ache. Her mother was surprised but tried not to overreact and accepted Gina's under-reaction.

I noted that I thought that Gina was gaining power. I asked Gina to do a sand scene called 'gaining power'. I attempted here to increase Gina's mindsight by assisting her to create a more elaborate mindsight map (Siegel, 1999). The most significant action taken in this scene was that all original characters that were small and scared or small helpers were changed to be physically 'bigger' versions of themselves. For example, Gina stated that the trickster is 'losing power' and replaced him with a small dinosaur. Gina also said she felt sorry for him and so added a couple of little helpers for him on his side. Her side remained bigger and more powerful. If all the figures in the tray represent parts of the self as Jung (1961) suggests, then Gina's empathy for a dark or negative part of the self was revealed by her adding helpers for the aggressive, attacking part of self. It may also be a way for Gina to re-configure feeling states, and provide some order, balance and control.

During the 'gaining power' scene I discovered that the wizard had now found the power stone 'because he knew the cat and girl were breaking down', as Gina said. These symbols were intermittently referred to as herself. During the next two sessions other forms of differentiation occurred, with Gina's verbalization that the scared cat and sad girl (originally chosen as fear and sad feeling state representations) no longer needed protection, rather they needed support. There was an emerging verbal awareness that although caring characters surrounded her, she does not need the same level of protection that was demonstrated earlier.

A number of distinct but simultaneous things appeared to emerge for Gina including: her self-knowledge that she had been overprotected by loved ones; the I-self referred to the Me-self that she will survive negative things; differentiation of 'like experiences' through the use of multiple characters over a number of sessions; integration through generalizations of becoming braver (a form of a trait label); and an actual behavioural change related to decreased stomach aches and a decreased fear of throwing up.

Conclusion

In summary, it would appear that the use of miniatures in sandplay offered Gina an experience of illuminating important elements of a 'Me map' (Siegel 1999). Through the power of play, Gina was able to tolerate and integrate new ideas related to the self. An emerging consciousness was observed through the self-awareness of having been over-protected by those around her. Gina claimed she really needed support versus protection. Her developmental growth was obvious as she was able to begin to self-regulate and gain control over a previously overwhelming problem of fear of throwing up. Gina was now more prepared to move from late childhood to an early adolescence phase of development and she returned to a previous normative level of functioning.

Key points

1. Through a case example, the play therapy process is examined using the dimension of consciousness.
2. The two primary dimensions, consciousness and directiveness, are illustrated through the theoretical construct – the Play Therapy Dimensions Model.
3. The chapter highlights that play therapists consider working in an intentional manner by observing indicators of the emergence of consciousness through the I-self, Me-self (developmental theory).
4. The case example of Gina captures the moment-to-moment movement along the consciousness dimension and the accompanying decision-making of the play therapist.

References

Baddeley, A. (1992). Working memory. *Science*, 255, pp. 556–9.
Beutler, L. E. and Clarkin, J. F. (1990). *Systematic treatment selection: Toward targeted therapeutic interventions*. Philadelphia, PS: Bruner/Mazel.
Chalmers, D. (2005). 'I'm conscious: He's just a zombie.' In S. Blackmore (ed.) *Conversations on consciousness* (pp. 36–9). Oxford: Oxford University Press.
Damasio, A. (1999). *The feeling of what happens: Body and emotions in the making of consciousness*. New York: Harcourt, Inc.
Dennett, D. C. (1991). *Consciousness explained*. Boston: Little, Brown.
Ellenberger, H. F. (1970). *The discovery of the unconscious: The history and evolution of dynamic psychiatry*. New York: Basic Books.
Gigerenzer, G. (2001). The adaptive toolbox. In G. Gigerenzer and R. Selten (eds), *Bounded rationality: The adaptive toolbox* (pp. 37–50). Cambridge, MA: MIT Press.
Guerney, L. (2001). Child-centred play therapy. *International Journal of Play Therapy*, 10, 2, 13–31.
Harter, S. (2012). *The construction of the self: Developmental and sociocultural foundations* (2nd edn). New York: The Guilford Press.
James, W. (1890). *Principles of psychology*. Chicago: Encyclopedia Britannica.
Jung, C. G. (1961). *Memories, dreams, reflections*. New York: Random House, Inc.

Kottman, T. (2003). *Partners in play: An Adlerian approach to play therapy* (2nd edn). Alexandria, VA: American Counselling Association.

Landreth, G. (2002). *Play Therapy: The art of the relationship* (2nd edn). Philadelphia, PA: Brunner/Routledge.

O'Connor, K. J. (2000). *The play therapy primer* (2nd edn). New York: John Wiley and Sons, Inc.

O'Connor, K. J. and Braverman, L. D. (eds) (2009). *Play therapy theory and practice: Comparing theories and techniques* (2nd edn). Hoboken, NJ: John Wiley and Sons, Inc.

Schottenbauer, M., Glass, C. R. and Arnkoff, D. B. (2007). Decision-making and psychotherapy integration: Theoretical considerations, preliminary data, and implications for future research. *Journal of Psychotherapy Integration* 17, 3, 225–50.

Siegel, D. J. (1999). *The developing mind: Toward a neurobiology of interpersonal experience*. New York: The Guilford Press.

Street, L. L., Niederehe, G. and Lebowitz, B. D. (2000). Toward greater public health relevance for psychotherapeutic intervention research: An NIMH workshop report. *Clinical Psychology: Science and Practice* 17, 2, 127–37.

VanFleet, R., Sywulak, A. and Sniscak, C. (2010). *Child-centred play therapy*. New York: Guilford.

Wachtel, P. L. (1977). *Psychoanalysis and Behavior Therapy: Towards an integration*. New York: Basic Books.

Wilson, K. and Ryan, V. (2005). *Play therapy: A non-directive approach for children and adolescents* (2nd edn). Oxford: Balliere Tindall.

Yasenik, L. and Gardner, K. (2012). *Play Therapy Dimensions Model: A Decision-Making Guide for Integrative Play Therapists*. London and Philadelphia: Jessica Kingsley Publishers.

Zelazo, P. D. (2004). The development of conscious control in childhood. *Trends in Cognitive Sciences*, 8, 12–17.

3 Using play therapeutically with children in a hospital setting

Lisa Morgan and Justine Howard

This chapter will demonstrate the invaluable role of play in supporting children's emotional health and well-being in a medical environment. The chapter will demonstrate that using appropriate techniques and carefully selected play materials can normalise the clinical environment and enable children to gain a sense of autonomy and control in a potentially distressing and unfamiliar situation. First we will consider how simply experiencing familiar play can increase resilience and reduce the distress of illness and admission to hospital. The chapter will then focus on therapeutic interventions such as preparation for theatre using puppets; distraction techniques such as bubble blowing and music; the post-operative value of using dreamsheets and stories; and games to encourage medical compliance. The theoretical underpinnings of these therapeutic techniques, and examples demonstrating their beneficial effects, will be included.

The clinical environment

Whilst the best place for an unwell child is often within the comfort of their own home (Save the Children Fund, 1989), there are times when hospitalisation cannot be avoided. One of the most important functions of play in a clinical setting is to normalise the environment, reducing the anxiety associated with fear of the unknown (Graham and Reynolds, 2013). Providing appropriate play activities can help children to frame their illness and hospital admission more positively. A hospital environment is very different to any environment a child is likely to have experienced before. The buildings themselves are often large, imposing and hard to navigate, with multiple corridors which all appear similar. The child will be surrounded by unfamiliar people in unfamiliar uniforms. Some wards may be quiet and calm with minimal activity whilst others might be noisy, busy places. Both of these are extremes by comparison to a child's experience of activity in their other life contexts. In addition, material differences in the environment are likely to be noticed – for example, the coldness of linoleum flooring, the uniform metal bed frames and plain linen, the curtained bed areas and the range of medical equipment either in use or ready for use. In order to create a sense of normality and reduce the potential anxiety caused by the starkness of the clinical environment, extraordinary effort is often put into the decoration and organisation of children's wards. Mobiles and pictures can be used to brighten up the clinical setting; however, these must be laminated so that they can be wiped regularly in accordance with infection control regulations.

The role of play in the clinical environment

Qualified play staff within paediatric departments are valuable team members. Their role involves ensuring that children's play needs are met from recreational, therapeutic and developmental perspectives. These three facets of hospital play provision will be the focus of this chapter. In addition however, hospitalisation can impact upon the whole family; as the child becomes distressed so in turn might their parents, siblings or other carers. A significant role of the play team is to support and spend time with the family; often this can just be a listening ear or providing reassurance about procedures or routines (Ellerton and Merriam 1994).

Recreational play

Normal play in hospital facilitates the continuation of physical, emotional, social and intellectual development. Playing with toys that are familiar can help children relax and bring a 'welcome relief from all the strange sights, smells, and bodily discomforts' (Lansdown and Goldman, 1988, p. 557). When confronted with the unfamiliar surroundings of the hospital ward, play activities reduce anxiety and enable children to gain control over their feelings and provide a safe outlet for them to express any fears and anxieties (McClowry and McLeod, 1990). The trauma of medical procedures or illness can take children out of their natural playful state into one of logic and reasoning (Deacon and Abramowitz, 2005). Their natural disposition towards play can be inhibited and so encouragement is vital. Planned play provision might of necessity be at the bedside for some or all of a child's stay. Daily activities in a playroom away from the ward, however, encourage children to move around and can increase levels of spontaneous play. Play can help children regain their confidence by socialising with other children and interacting with play staff, which in turn makes them feel comfortable and less frightened (Department of Health, 2003). Having a structured play timetable (see the example in Table 3.1) is also important so that children have a sense of routine and are able to take some control over planning what they would like to do. This small sense of autonomy is particularly important when, for much of their hospital stay, procedures and routine are largely out of the child's control (Lingnell and Dunn, 1999).

The aim of the playroom is to create an inviting, child friendly environment. Play materials are carefully selected, taking into consideration the needs of the many different ages and medical needs of the children admitted. A wide variety of toys are provided – for example, sensory play, pretend play and role play materials, art and craft activities along with play which involves music or movement. There are limitations to the types of materials which can be provided, however, due to health and safety regulations; toys routinely available must be durable enough to withstand daily cleaning. Other materials such as playdough or plasticine can be offered in small quantities in containers labelled for each individual child to ensure infection control. Soft toys are not made available for these reasons; however, children will often bring in such comfort items from home. For other items we might wish to use for sensory or mark making play (e.g. cornflour goo or shaving foam) we seek advice from the pharmacy department for potential allergy issues.

Educational and developmental

Children who have been in hospital long term may have specific play needs. This might also apply to the chronically ill child who regularly visits the hospital for treatment. The developmental play needs of these children can be different as they may have had to endure more invasive procedures or deal with ongoing medication. Here, individual play plans are designed to meet care and developmental needs through one to one therapeutic play sessions (Frankenfield, 1996). For children who are unable to attend the playroom, stimulating hand and eye co-ordination using appropriate play materials such as building blocks and threading toys at the bedside can promote their fine manipulative skills. For children who have been bed bound from birth, the core muscles of their abdomen may be under-developed and activities which encourage reaching or sitting up for short periods will promote muscular development. Sensory materials such as tactile toys with music

Table 3.1 Example of a structured play timetable

Monday	Tuesday	Wednesday	Thursday	Friday
8.00–Breakfast	8.00–Breakfast	8.00–Breakfast	8.00–Breakfast	8.00–Breakfast
8.30–10.00 Colouring and free play	8.30–10.00 Colouring and free play	8.30–10.00 Colouring and free play	8.30–10.00 Colouring and free play	8.30–10.00 Colouring and free play
10.00–11.00 Gluing and Sticking activity	10.00–11.00 Chalking	10.00–11.00 Gluing and Sticking activity	10.00–11.00 Scratch Art/stencilling	10.00–11.00 Gluing and Sticking activity
1.00–2.00 Painting	1.00–2.00 Painting	1.00–2.00 Painting	1.00–2.00 Painting	1.00–2.00 Painting
3.30–4.30 Board games challenge	3.30–4.30 Quiz Time!	3.00–4.30 Midweek Movie Mania!	3.30–4.30 Story time or Music time	3.30–4.30 Bingo Bonanza
5.00–Tea Time	5.00–Tea Time	5.00–Tea Time	5.00–Tea Time	5.00–Tea Time
5.30–6.45 Colouring and free play	5.30–6.45 Colouring and free play	5.30–6.45 Colouring and free play	5.30–6.45 Colouring and free play	5.30–6.45 Colouring and free play

or vibration can stimulate a child's senses. When considering a child's play needs it is important to recognise the way in which play develops over time and how earlier forms of play lay the foundations for the following stages. Jennings' (1999) Embodiment, Projection and Role approach is a useful model here. Embodiment play helps children learn about their physical self and the fact that they exist as separate to others or their environment. Once this is learned, children are able to play with objects outside of the self – for example, using one thing to stand for another in pretend play. With an increased ability for abstract thought, children can then progress to more elaborate role play and drama. This pattern of play development is consistent with the development of the brain discussed in Chapter 11.

Case study

Thomas was born with a stomach problem and has spent all 11 months of his life in hospital undergoing surgery and intensive treatments. Thomas's family live quite a distance from the hospital and family and work demands have prevented them from being at his bedside as frequently as they would wish. The opportunity to develop secure attachment bonds during the early months of life has been limited for Thomas and the nature of his condition has meant holding and cuddling him could be awkward. Now that he is stronger and no longer reliant on static medical equipment, Thomas enjoys being held and carried around the ward by staff. However, he cries immediately, and for lengthy periods, on being put down. Whereas when he was very ill he was sleepy, he has now become more alert and aware of his environment.

Our play plan for Thomas involved regular periods of holding, eye-to-eye contact and games such as peek a boo. Our aim was for Thomas to establish a sense of trust in his relationships with the adults around him. We also planned play with a variety of sensory toys so that Thomas could develop more body awareness. Finally, in relation to his physical development, as Thomas had been lying sedentary in his cot for a prolonged period, there was a need to promote play activities which encouraged reaching out and sitting up, in order to develop core muscle strength.

We have seen many benefits from this programme. Thomas has built positive relationships with the nursing staff and regular visits to the playroom have promoted social skills. He no longer cries so persistently when he is put down and seems generally happier in himself, enjoying the sensory stimulation we have provided in play sessions and around his cot area. Playing, talking, and singing have encouraged Thomas to interact with others by smiling, cooing and laughing. He is also now able to sit up with the aid of a back support for short periods. Thomas's care and play needs will be reviewed when he is due to leave the hospital and care will continue via a play specialist within the community health team.

Therapeutic play

Play can serve a variety of therapeutic functions in a hospital environment. It can be used as a means of preparing children for surgery or medical procedures; as a means of distraction during uncomfortable or painful procedures; or as a way of encouraging children to comply with their drug or physical exercise plans.

Play preparation

Play based techniques are highly effective in preparing children for surgery (O'Conner-Von, 2000; Li and Lopez, 2008). As well as talking to children about their illness and medical care, incorporating the use of puppets and dolls can decrease anxiety and prepare children effectively for procedures (Zahr 1998). Used for modelling purposes, we can encourage children to copy the puppet in exploring, touching, and practising using the medical equipment prior to their operation (Alger *et al.* 1985). Creating a character that the child can focus on, in a fun and playful manner, can build trust and provide reassurance. Puppets can be used spontaneously during ward rounds to find out how children are feeling as talking to the puppet can be easier than talking to the medical staff (Athanassiadou *et al.* 2009). They can also be used in structured preparation techniques.

> As a paediatric nurse working on the surgical ward, I can't emphasise enough how important I feel play preparation is for the child. What is normal for staff must be so frightening for the child and family. Play preparation makes the nurse's job easier...patients are happy, relaxed, and prepared....We have a whole puppet family now and they are loved by all of the children.
>
> Paediatric Nurse, day surgery ward

Case study – an example of play preparation using 'Boris'

Molly was four years old and had been admitted into hospital for the insertion of grommets. On admission to the ward it was evident that Molly was unsure of the environment and appeared quiet and apprehensive. I introduced myself to Molly and her mum as the toy nurse, and immediately she smiled with curiosity.

I use a child living puppet as the children relate to it well and it has a gloved hand which I can use as my own. I also use a decorated box containing surgical items relevant to the child's procedure such as venflons (the tube which is inserted into the back of the hand for drug administration), breathing masks or dressings. I call the box a 'tap tap box' as through the preparation process, I ask the children to tap the box to make it open.

I offered Molly and her mum the opportunity for me to explain the procedure to Molly using play as a means of communication. I told Molly that I had a very special friend called Boris who would like to meet her to show her our hospital 'butterflies' and 'mermaid masks'. Molly was excited, yet I could sense that she was still anxious. I returned to Molly's bedside with Boris and my 'tap tap box' which was filled with venflons (butterflies) and breathing masks (mermaid masks).

'Hello Molly, this is Boris. Would you like to shake his hand?' Molly smiled and reached out to touch Boris. 'What is in the box?' she asked. 'Shall we sing Boris's "tap tap" song and then we can open it?' 'Yes, yes,' Molly shouted.

I began to sing the 'tap tap' song as Molly and Boris tapped the top of the box rhythmically. When we had finished singing, Molly eagerly opened the box and removed the lid. She pulled out the breathing mask and handed it to me. I asked Molly if she knew why she had come into hospital and she told me the doctors were going to make her ears better but that she would have to go to sleep.

I said this was true and asked Molly what she would like to dream of whilst she was having her special sleep. 'I want to dream of being a princess,' she answered. 'That's great,' I replied. 'To help you go to sleep for your magic dream we need to see the special hospital equipment. Do you think that you could pretend to be the mermaid swimming in the sea by blowing up the balloon at the end of the mask? Shall we see if Boris can do it first?' Molly said yes and held the end of the mask in her hand.

'This is our mermaid mask," I said, placing it over Boris's face. I made Boris try to blow up the mask. '1, 2, 3. Oh no, Boris couldn't do it. Shall we see if you can?' Molly quickly placed the mask over her face and began to blow into it. As the balloon began to inflate Molly began to blow faster and faster. 'I can do it,' she said, smiling proudly to herself. Boris moved closer and Molly reached out to hug him. 'Well done, you're just like a mermaid swimming with the dolphins under the sea,' I told her. 'Now shall we see our hospital butterflies that the doctors use to help send us for our magic dreams?' Boris looked inside the box and pulled out one of the venflons. 'This is our hospital butterfly,' I said, as I began to fly it around in the air landing it on Boris's arm. 'Shall we pretend that your hand is like a flower where the butterfly can land?'

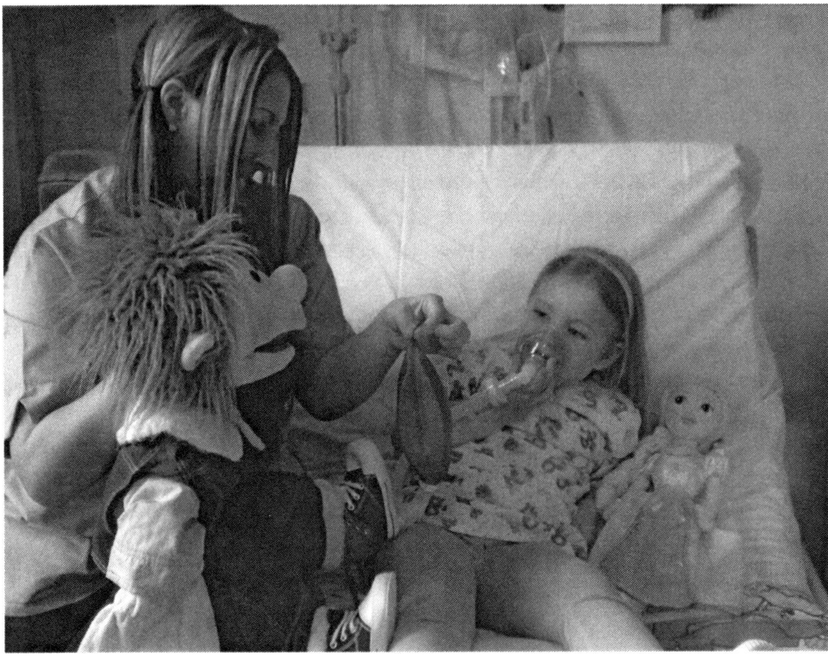

Figure 3.1 Play specialist using the puppet, Boris, with a child

Molly replied, 'Yes. please' holding out her arm in front of him. 'Will it hurt when the doctors land it on my hand?' she asked me. 'The nurses will put some magic cream on the back of your hand which will make your hand feel tingly and then the butterfly will have a soft landing,' I reassured Molly. Molly seemed content with what I had told her and began to fly the butterfly in the air and landed it on her teddy. 'I like Boris,' Molly said as she reached over and touched him. 'Can he come with me when I go to see the doctor?' 'Of course,' I assured her. 'You can show the doctor how clever you are at blowing up the balloon and tell them what you're going to dream of when you're having your magic sleep.' Molly was excited about her adventure to theatre and her special dream. She put the mask and venflon back into the box and I took Molly and her mum to visit the playroom where Molly played until it was her turn for her operation.

Tailoring the approach for each child, accounting for their likes and dislikes, makes the preparation personal and meaningful, helping the child to feel safe and in control. Preparation for theatre or procedures like having a blood test are often the first stage of the child's hospital journey. Providing children with an opportunity to handle the medical equipment using puppets as their ally and model facilitates understanding. The opportunity to talk encourages children to plan their own hospital adventure, creating their own 'special dream'.

Accompanying the child on their journey to the anaesthetic room enables preparation to blend with distraction techniques to further alleviate anxiety. Inside the anaesthetic room the play specialist works in partnership with the nurses and anaesthetists to ensure that the child remains as calm and comfortable as possible. Distraction techniques and encouraging the child to imagine their 'special dream' enhances positive framing and allows the child to blend fantasy with reality (Herron and Sutton Smith, 1971). Children can be encouraged to talk about the dream they have had on their return to the ward following their procedure using dream sheets (see Figure 3.2). Even if they haven't actually dreamt what it was they thought they would or they decide to draw or write about something different on their 'dream sheet', merely talking about the process encourages them to come to terms with their procedure.

> As a paediatric nurse and ward manager, my experience of working with children spans over 38 years...children and play go hand in hand... children who are well prepared for theatre using play can be calmer and embrace the experience, whilst children who have had no play preparation are often worried and afraid.
>
> Paediatric Sister and Ward Manager

Distraction techniques
Distraction techniques can help children suffering from the anxiety caused by medical procedures to gain control over their feelings (Sylva and Stein, 1990). Whilst this type of play is beneficial in helping a child get through a necessary painful procedure, however, it is important that they remain aware and understand what is going to happen to them (Harvey, 1984). Developmentally appropriate interventions work in partnership with preparation techniques, helping to support and alleviate any panic and distress. Distraction techniques are not used as a tool for tricking the child but as a means of refocusing the child's attention, enabling procedures to go as smoothly as possible (Lansdown, 1992).

Useful distraction techniques for younger children:
- Bubbles – these can be one of the most effective mesmerising distraction techniques for younger children, using a fairy or princess wand, a puppet to 'pop' the bubbles or letting the child 'catch' them in their hands.
- Books – musical, pop up and sensory books work well with younger children as they provide a variety of things to focus upon.
- Music and singing – listening to nursery rhymes reassures and calms, especially if this is something the child is familiar with in their home environment.

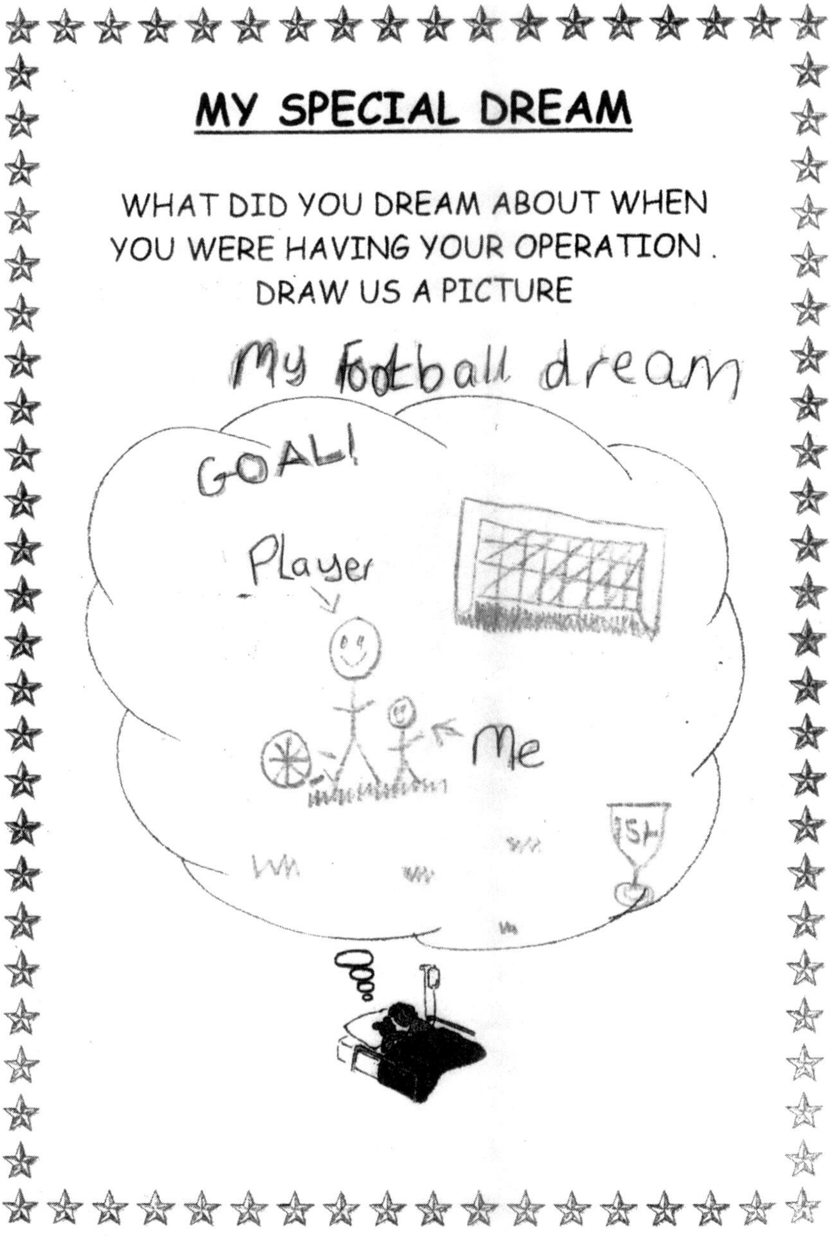

Figure 3.2 Example of a completed dream sheet picture

MY HOSPITAL ADVENTURE

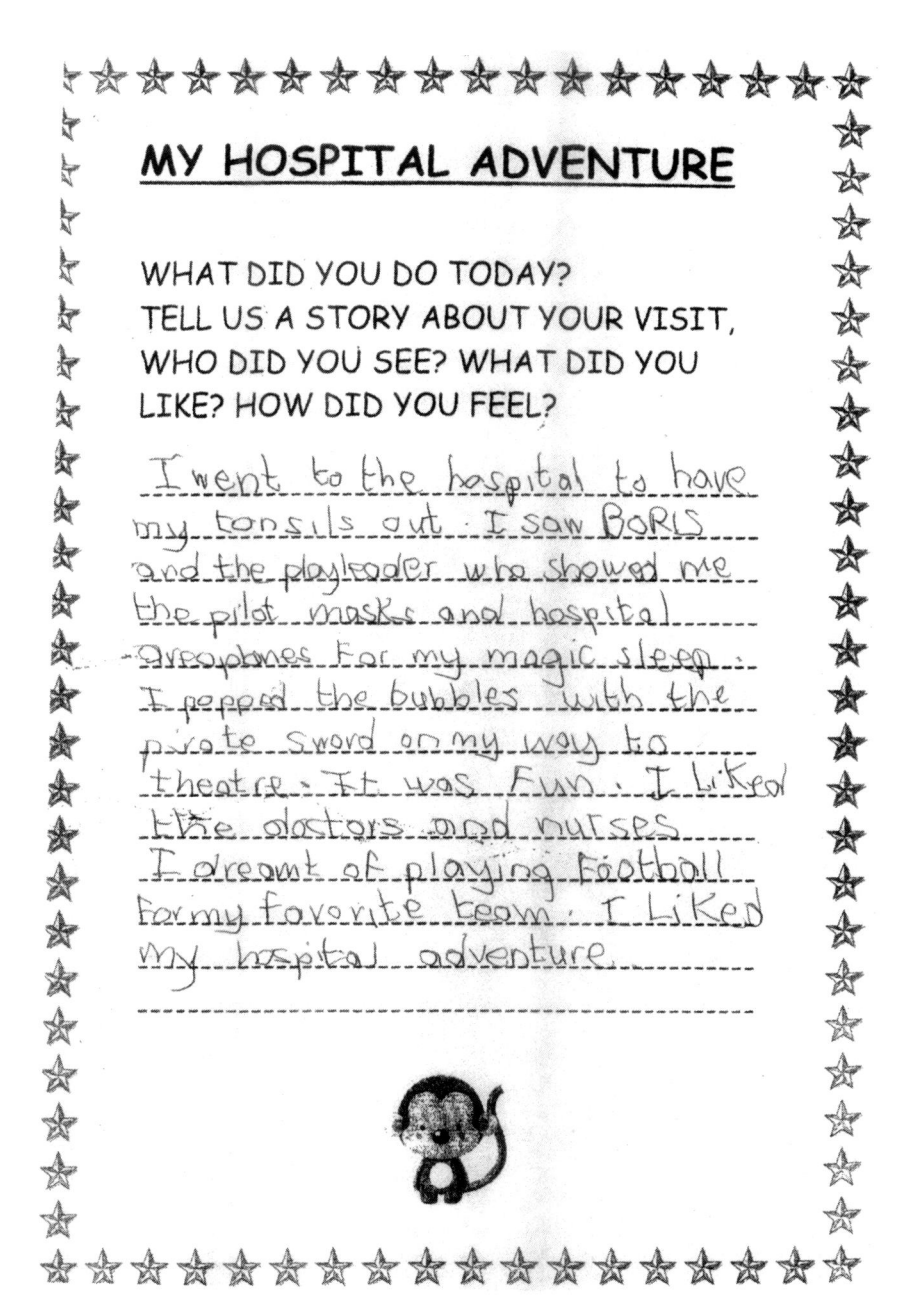

WHAT DID YOU DO TODAY?
TELL US A STORY ABOUT YOUR VISIT,
WHO DID YOU SEE? WHAT DID YOU
LIKE? HOW DID YOU FEEL?

I went to the hospital to have my tonsils out. I saw BORIS and the playleader who showed me the pilot masks and hospital aeroplanes for my magic sleep. I popped the bubbles with the pirate sword on my way to theatre. It was fun. I liked the doctors and nurses. I dreamt of playing football for my favorite team. I liked my hospital adventure.

Figure 3.3 Example of a dream sheet story

- Touch toys – light up and musical touch toys can provide instant distraction as the child is actively engaged in the activity.
- Electronic devices – pre-loaded with children's favourite cartoons, these can also be useful as they are familiar to the child.

Useful distraction techniques with older children:
- Games and puzzles – older children find using a hand held game or play station a preferred choice of distraction.
- Controlled breathing – encouraging the child to imagine that they are blowing up an imaginary balloon or a feather up into the air works well to help concentrate on their breathing, instantly calming them.
- Visualization – encouraging the child to think of something special to them, such as a pet or a favourite toy can help them to feel in a safe space.
- Guided imagery – here we might talk to the child about something they would love to do, like going to a pop concert, swimming with dolphins or walking on the beach. We might ask questions like 'What can you see?' 'Who is on the beach with you?' 'Is the sun shining?'
- Talking through the procedure with older children or teenagers about things that interest them can sometimes be all that is needed to distract them. However, this will be based on our assessment of the child's anxiety.

Post-procedural play

Post-procedural play can be a useful means of identifying any fears or misconceptions a child may have following a treatment or procedure. It can also help to identify a child's play needs. Effective communication is crucial to the perioperative care process and children's natural form of communication is through play (Wennstrom *et al.* 2008). Using play to normalise the environment and to prepare the child for surgery have already supported the development of a trusting relationship that encourages questioning and openness. Post-procedural play enables the child to further work through the events they have experienced and move forward toward recovery. Some children can be reluctant to comply with their treatments – for example, not wanting to take their medicines or do their physiotherapy exercises. Play input here can ensure that they follow their medical care plan without feeling forced or under pressure (Ispa *et al.* 1988). At a basic level, personalised 'star charts' can be an effective method of encouragement in taking medicines. However, playing games that the children relate to and are actively involved in are particularly successful, for example:

- 'Barbie or superhero' picnics on the bed – placing the child's favourite figures on the bed and having small plates of the child's favourite foods

laid out as a picnic can help encourage the child to eat. If puppets were used during preparation, then involving them in a picnic can also be successful as the child is familiar with them as a play partner
- 'Bush tucker trials' – we noticed that the older children on the ward loved the television programme 'I'm a celebrity get me out of here'. The programme involves bush tucker trials where contestants are dared to eat unusual foods in the jungle! We fill medicine pots with foods such as jelly, toast, biscuit, yoghurt or milkshake. Children compete with one another to complete their trials, winning stars for their wards.

Individual referrals

Requests for the play specialist to see individual children might be made by doctors or other members of the multi-disciplinary care team. These might be made, for example, for children who are needle phobic, frightened of a hospital admission, suffer with an eating disorder or have a chronic illness such as cystic fibrosis or diabetes. Where possible, setting up agreed meeting times with planned aims and objectives alongside the child, allows them to gain a sense of control over what is happening and using play to promote their health care and development means they can move forward at their own pace (Gariepy and Howe, 2003). Howard and McInnes (2013) describe the various ways in which some diagnosed disabilities can impact on children's play behaviour. For example, a child with cerebral palsy may have movement and co-ordination difficulties, impacting on the development of their early sensory play skills and general confidence in playing. Here our focus might be on encouraging a sense of control using toys that demonstrate cause and effect, developing self-esteem. The number of sessions held will depend on the nature of the issue. For individual referrals, any therapeutic intervention will be planned according to the child's medical case history and using as much information as possible about the child's own likes, dislikes or patterns of play behaviour.

Case study

Annie is 13 years old and suffers from needle phobia, after failing to receive her injections in school. Annie was referred to me for therapeutic play intervention. I contacted her mum and we set up a convenient time for them to visit me at the hospital. During our first session we talked about Annie's previous experiences and fears. We also spent time talking about school, friends, hobbies, likes and dislikes. We made a plan for the next session a week later and asked Annie to write down any thoughts that she had during the week and to bring them with her to the next session.

Our next session involved looking at some of the different types of needles that could be used for injections. I applied some 'magic cream' to the back of one of Annie's hands which we had talked about in our previous meeting, so that at the end of the session she could test how well it numbed the area. I laid out a variety of syringes (with no needles attached) so that Annie could engage in handling them if she showed an interest in doing so. Annie was keen to touch them and held them in her hand very calmly. This was a good first step in familiarising her with the equipment. Throughout the session Annie carefully examined the materials. Once the cream was removed, Annie used the venflon to press on the back of her hand. She was pleasantly surprised how it felt, comparing it to the different feeling she got when she pressed the venflon to the other hand. Throughout the rest of the session Annie continued to handle the equipment confidently and was very pleased with herself on her progress.

Session three began by applying cream again to the back of Annie's hand to reinforce how effective it was at numbing the area. This time we were going to see if Annie could handle the venflons with the needles still inside (tips initially covered). I laid out a tray with the venflon, a glove with water and an orange. I showed Annie the tip of the needle for her to see just how small it was. I began to demonstrate how easily the needle pierced through the glove and the orange without any force or pressure.

Annie was keen to try this herself. She pierced the orange and was surprised how easily it went in. She did the same thing with the glove and was amazed that such a tiny hole had been pierced. Annie used the needle to pierce the orange and the glove several times over. Annie wanted to test how numb her hand was again and so we took a new venflon without a needle attached and she touch the back of her hand, repetitively and with increased vigour. She was amazed not to be able to feel it. She seemed very proud of herself and said she wanted to try to see if she could have her injection again. We discussed what we were going to visualize and think about during the injection.

I met Annie when she arrived at the hospital and, after already applying her cream at home, she was ready. It was evident that Annie was still a little anxious and frightened as the nurse was about to proceed, however with some deep breathing exercises and recanting our preparation sessions, Annie had the injection. Afterwards she said, 'I never felt it'. She was so pleased with herself, she cried with delight.

Conclusion

Therapeutic play has an invaluable role in a hospital setting in relation to a child's emotional health, medical care, holistic development and successful recovery. It can significantly improve the hospital experience for children. Play reduces anxiety in the child and also their family members and/or care givers (Fincher *et al.* 2012). Current research clearly demonstrates the value of play preparation techniques for the reduction of stress and anxiety, and post-procedural play for children's speedy recovery and treatment compliance. In addition, research clearly demonstrates that children who are well prepared before treatment suffer less anxiety and return to health more speedily than those who are not (LaMontagne *et al.* 1996). With the current pressures on the National Health System, staff are having to multi-task in their roles. However, it is vital that we continue to recognise the role of the hospital play team in meeting children's recreational, developmental and therapeutic play needs. Play can aid recovery, promote healing and reduce any long term psychological effects of sickness or hospitalisation. Play in hospital reduces the potential for long term effects because it offers children freedom, control, and autonomy (Lingnell and Dunn, 1999).

Within the paediatric health care system, our central goal is to ensure the emotional and physical well-being of children. Therapeutic play can offer long term benefits by fostering positive framing in relation to medical experiences. Whether the play is directive or non-directive, children can express feelings related to fear and anxiety (Le Vieux, 1999). Play is a child's natural mode of action and inherently builds confidence, esteem and resiliency (Fearn and Howard, 2011). Spending quality time with children and their families, participating in play activities that can be enjoyed in spite of illness, enables the child to achieve a sense of control over what can be a potentially frightening experience. Therapeutic play focuses on the process of play as a coping mechanism for children to master adverse experiences such as hospitalisation. Children themselves have described play as their best method of coping, when they are ill or in hospital (Salmela *et al.* 2010).

Key points

Play delivered by a dedicated team of well-trained specialists can serve multiple functions within the clinical environment, notably:-

1. It normalises the clinical environment and enables children to continue with familiar aspects of their daily lives in spite of illness.
2. It can be a useful distraction technique during painful or unfamiliar procedures.

3. It enables children to work through and talk about any worries or concerns they have about their illness or medical care.
4. It can provide a means of communicating key information to children about medical procedures, ensuring they are comfortable and aware of what is going to happen.
5. It can be used to support post-procedural care and compliance with drug or physical therapy regimes.

References

Alger, I., Linn, S. and Beardslee, W. (1985). Puppetry as a therapeutic tool for hospitalized children. *Hospital and Community Psychiatry*, 36(2), 129–130.

Athanassiadou, E., Tsiantis, J., Christogiorgos, S. and Kolaitis, G. (2009). Evaluation of the effectiveness of psychological preparation of children for minor surgery by puppet play and brief mother counselling. *Psychotherapy and Psychosomatics*, 78: 62–63.

Deacon, B. and Abramowitz, J. (2005). Patients' perceptions of pharmacological and cognitive-behavioral treatments for anxiety disorders. *Behaviour Therapy*, 36(2), 139–145.

Department of Health (1991). *The Welfare of Children and Young People in Hospital*. London: HMSO.

Ellerton, M.-L., and Merriam, C, (1994). Preparing children and families psychologically for day surgery: an evaluation. *Journal of Advanced Nursing*, 19, 1057–1062.

Fearn, M. and Howard, J. (2011). Play as a resource for children facing adversity. *Children and Society*, 26(6), pp. 456–468.

Fincher, W., Shaw, J. and Ramelet, A. (2013). The effectiveness of a standardised preoperative preparation in reducing child and parent anxiety: a single-blind randomised controlled trial. *Journal of Clinical Nursing*, 7–8, pp. 946–955.

Frankenfield, P. (1996). The power of humor and play as a nursing intervention for a child with cancer: A case report. *Journal of Pediatric Oncology Nursing*, 13(1), 15–20.

Gariepy, N. and Howe, N. (2003). The therapeutic power of play: examining the play of young children with leukemia. *Child: Care, Health, and Development*, 29(6), pp. 523–537.

Graham, P. and Reynolds, S. (2013). *Cognitive Behaviour Therapy for Children and Families*. Cambridge: CUP.

Harvey, S. (1984). Training the hospital play specialist. *Early Child Development and Care*, 17, pp. 227–290.

Herron, R. E. and Sutton-Smith, B. (1971). *Child's Play*. New York: Wiley.

Howard, J. and McInnes, K. (2013). *The Essence of Play*. Routledge: London.

Ispa, J., Barrett, B. and Kim, Y. (1988). Effects of supervised play in a hospital waiting room. *Children's Health Care*, 16(3), pp. 195–200.

Jennings, S. (1999). *Introduction to Developmental Playtherapy.* London: Jessica Kingsley Publishers Ltd.

LaMontagne, L. L., Hepworth, J. T., Johnson, B. D. and Cohen, F. (1996). Children's preoperative coping and its effect on postoperative anxiety and return to normal activity. *Nursing Research*, 45(3), pp. 141–147.

Lansdown, R. (1992). The psychological health status of children in hospital. *Journal of the Royal Society of Medicine*, 85, pp. 125–126.

Lansdown, R. and Goldman, A. (1988). The psychological care of children with malignant disease. *Journal of Child Psychology and Psychiatry.* 29, pp. 555–567.

Le Vieux, J. (1999). Group play therapy with grieving children. In D. S. Sweeney and L. E. Homeyer (eds), *The handbook of group play therapy: How to do it, how it works, whom it's best for* (pp. 375–388). San Francisco, CA: Jossey-Bass.

Li, H. C. W. and Lopez, V. (2008). Effectiveness and appropriateness of therapeutic play intervention in preparing children for surgery: a randomized controlled trial study. *Journal for Specialists in Paediatric Nursing*, 13(2), pp. 63–73.

Lingnell, L. and Dunn, L. (1999). Group play therapy: wholeness and healing for the hospitalized child. In D. S. Sweeney and L. E. Homeyer (eds), *The handbook of group play therapy: How to do it, how it works, whom it's best for* (pp. 359–374). San Francisco, CA: Jossey-Bass.

McClowry, S. G. and McLeod, S. M. (1990). The psychological responses of school age children to hospitalisation. *Children's Health Care*, 19(3), pp. 155–161.

O'Conner-Von, S. (2000). Preparing children for surgery: an integrative research review. *AORN Journal*, 71(2), pp. 334–343.

Salmela, M., Salantera, S., Ruotsalainen, T. and Aronen, E. (2010). Coping strategies for hospital-related fears in pre-school-aged children. *Journal of Pediatrics and Child Health*, 46(3), pp. 108–114.

Save the Children Fund (1989). *Hospital: A deprived environment for children? The case for hospital play schemes.* London: Save the Children.

Sylva, K. and Stein, A. (1990). Effects of hospitalisation on young children. *Child Psychology and Psychiatry Newsletter*, 12(1), pp. 3–8.

Wennstrom, B., Hallberg, L. and Bergh, I. (2008). Use of perioperative dialogues with children undergoing day surgery. *Journal of Advanced Nursing*, 62(1), pp. 96–106.

Zahr, L. K. (1998). Therapeutic play for hospitalised pre-schoolers in Lebanon. *Paediatric Nursing*, 24, pp. 449–454.

4

Therapeutic play as an intervention for children exposed to domestic violence

Trish Gettins

Introduction

There has been a growing awareness of the scale of domestic violence and the devastating impact this can have on children. Domestic violence is an increasing public, policy and political concern. Research surrounding the experiences of children's service practitioners, family members and children's own accounts all demonstrate that domestic violence has a significant impact on the lives of children and on their current future well-being.

The UK Government defines domestic violence as

> any incident or pattern of incidents of controlling, coercive or threatening behaviour, violence or abuse between those aged 16 or over who are or have been intimate partners or family members regardless of gender or sexuality. This can encompass but is not limited to the following types of abuse: psychological, physical, sexual, financial and emotional.
>
> (Home Office, 2013).

Domestic violence accounts for 25 per cent of all reported crime within the UK with an estimated cost of £16 billion per year (10,000 Safer Lives Project, 2012; Walby, 2009). In 2011, 1354 children and young people fled to refuges across Wales due to dangerous levels of domestic violence in their home; however, support could only be offered to 330 of these (Thatcher, 2012). This chapter will focus on the various forms of domestic violence, its prevalence and impact on children, the services available to support children and, specifically, the value of play as a therapeutic tool.

The scope and prevalence of domestic violence

Within the UK it is estimated 750,000 children are exposed to domestic abuse each year. Organisations supporting children affected by domestic violence are often not core funded and there is a lack of consistency in terms of the level and types of support available (Thatcher, 2012). In November 2012, the Welsh Government put a White Paper out for consultation, outlining policy and legislative proposals aimed at ending violence against women, domestic abuse and sexual violence (Welsh Assembly Government, 2012). One of the recommendations from the White Paper is that domestic violence awareness should form part of the national curriculum within all educational settings across Wales; it has been made clear, however, that there are no additional funds to support this service.

In 90 per cent of domestic violence incidents a child is present or in the adjacent room (Department of Health, 2002). Neglect and domestic violence are closely linked and the causes of neglect are varied. Studies suggest that, amongst other things, parental mental health problems, substance misuse (Stone, 1998; Cleaver *et al.* 2007), domestic violence (Shepard and Raschick, 1999; Cawson, 2002), unemployment and poverty (Thoburn *et al.* 2000) are factors which increase the likelihood of neglect. Sadly, the issue is complicated by the fact that families often experience many of these issues simultaneously.

Neglect is the most common reason for children to be placed on the child protection register in Wales or be subject to a child protection plan in England (Bunting, 2011).

In a study of 139 serious case reviews in England 2009–2011, 63 per cent of cases were found to have domestic violence as a risk factor (Brandon *et al.* 2012). This study shows the devastating impact domestic violence can have on children and young people. Unstable and abusive relationships increase the risk of child neglect and abuse.

Research focusing specifically on the effects of neglect is still very limited. As neglect often co-exists with other forms of maltreatment, what we know about the effects of neglect is derived primarily from studies that examine neglect in conjunction with other forms of abuse. Chronic and severe forms of neglect pose a serious threat to a child's survival (Thatcher, 2012).

Glaser's (2000) review of work carried out in the fields of neuro-biology and developmental psychology showed that emotional neglect can have adverse effects on the development of a child's brain, having potentially devastating long-term effects for the child.

The impact of domestic violence on children's health and development

Studies show that children who witness abuse and live in a violent environment are at risk of serious behavioural and other psychological problems (Spilsbury *et al.* 2007). Rivett, Howard and Harold's (2006) findings suggest the children from homes with domestic violence show more aggression, display impaired cognitive and motor abilities and have delayed verbal development. Other studies confirm that a child witnessing domestic violence has negative effects on behavioural, psychological and emotional development (Huth-Bocks *et al.* 2001; Stover, 2005; Dowd *et al.* 2006; Ybarra *et al.* 2007). Children from homes of domestic violence are 60 per cent more likely to suffer physical and sexual abuse from the perpetrator (NSPCC, 2011).

The emotional, behavioural, physical, social and cognitive effects on children who have been exposed to domestic violence are summarised in Table 4.1.

It is important to recognise that not all children who witness domestic violence will exhibit the problems indicated above, or be subject to direct physical or sexual abuse themselves (Spilbury *et al.* 2007; Chiodo *et al.* 2008). Many children exposed to domestic violence show no greater problems than those who have not been exposed (Chiodo *et al.* 2008). Some children who are exposed to domestic violence face no greater risks than children who live in 'distressed' relationships without abuse (Dowd *et al.* 2006). A number of factors may influence the degree to which child witnesses are affected. They include the age of the child witness, gender, intellectual ability, socioeconomic status, level of social support, the quality of the child's relationship with the parents, the amount of time that has passed since the child's exposure to violence and the child's resilience (Dowd *et al.* 2006). It is clear however, that regardless of these differences, specialist tailored support is useful in helping them to overcome their experience.

From a practical perspective, it is important to find out exactly what each child has experienced and how they appear to be coping with these experiences – in order to gain an understanding of what the possible impact might be – rather than thinking in terms of a warning sign checklist. It can be hard to discern the specific impact of living with domestic violence on a child, especially as some of the resulting behaviours also occur in children experiencing other forms of abuse or neglect (Holden and Ritchie, 1991). For many children, the impact is compounded by the effects of the direct sexual and/or physical abuse they are also experiencing from the same abuser.

Table 4.1 The impact of exposure to domestic abuse across developmental domains

Emotional effects	Behavioural effects	Physical effects	Social effects	Cognitive effects
fear/insecurity	nervous/jumpy	eating disturbances	difficulty trusting	developmental delays
non-responsiveness	cries a lot	sleeping disturbances	problems relating to other children	learning delays
inconsolable	poor impulse control	developmental delays	social isolation	experience unclear and inconsistent boundaries
low self-esteem	regressive behaviour	psychosomatic disorders	blurred social boundaries	learn to blame others for one's own action
withdrawal	acting out violently	stress related illness	school problems	learn to equate love with abuse
anger	withdrawn	physical injuries	embarrassed about family	learn to disrespect
conflicted loyalties	difficulty in school	physical/sexual abuse	experience confusion about gender roles	learn perpetrating abuse is a way to get what you want
embarrassment	young carer			learn unrealistic cause and effect relationships
stress	adult affect			inability to empathise
difficulty trusting	overachiever			
guilt	running away			
shame	drug and alcohol use			
confusion	truancy			
feeling of responsibility	abusive in a dating relationship			
sadness	suicidal			
powerlessness				
depression				
suicidal				
emotional self-regulation				

Supporting children affected by domestic violence through play

There are many different services available to support children, young people and families who have experienced domestic violence; however, support for child witnesses often arrives too late, being remedial rather than preventative. Whilst the victims of abuse may receive immediate support via specialist counselling, support for the child witness can be secondary, offered through referral after the child is presenting with behavioural or emotional difficulties. As a therapeutic play specialist working with children exposed to domestic violence, my aim is to increase resilience and emotional health through the powers inherent in play, in order to reduce the potential impact of exposure. Therapeutic play at this preventative level can also facilitate referral to specialist support services, such as play therapy or counselling, at the earliest possible opportunity.

Play is essential for all children as it contributes to their social, physical, and cognitive development. Freud (1961) noted that, 'Every child at play behaves like an imaginative writer; in that he creates a world of his own, or more truly, he rearranges the things of his world and orders it in a new way which pleases him better' (cited in Levy, 2008, p. 282). Children gain an understanding of their thoughts and actions during play, develop the ability to regulate their behaviour and develop new skills (Tsao, 2002). Through play, children experience a sense of achievement which contributes greatly to self-esteem (Erikson, 1965). Arguably, the confidence and emotional strength gained through play acts as a springboard for development in all other domains (Howard and McInnes, 2013). For children dealing with adversity, the inherent power of play to increase resilience is of even greater importance (Fearn and Howard, 2011).

Children benefit from their own self-directed play experiences at the home and in school. Playworkers provide open access play opportunities for children in the community. Their focus is on children's right to play and the need for children to direct their own play experiences, wherever possible. Most of the open access play provided by playworkers is recreational. Play therapists work with children using play as a therapeutic medium for the identification, communication and resolution of emotional or behavioural issues. Their work is remedial in that their aim is to explicitly support children to resolve issues through the development of a therapeutic relationship. Therapeutic play specialists provide play sessions designed to enhance children's holistic development. They work with individuals and groups, facilitating play skills that promote well-being and resilience (Howard, 2009). The aim of the therapeutic play specialist within a domestic violence support service is to maximise the value of play at a preventative level, but also to identify any need for referral to specialist support services as early as possible.

Structured group play activities for children and young people who have been exposed to domestic violence

Children and young people need to be listened to, believed and supported. Children and young people are not usually looking for solutions for their worries and fears, but rather an opportunity to share these in a safe environment. Peled and Davies (1995) state that the main aims of group work for children and young people who have been exposed to domestic violence are:

- to gain an understanding of all that has happened to them
- to understand that living with domestic violence is not their fault
- to realise they are not alone and to share experiences
- to explore emotions and develop appropriate coping strategies
- to address the impact domestic violence has had on relationships in the family
- to work on feelings towards parents, including torn loyalties and conflicting emotions
- to build self-esteem, resilience and protective strategies for the future
- to have fun!

Examples of structured activities for group work with children

- 'The Huge Bag of Worries' written by Virginia Ironside (a story for children to help them address their worries)
  Read the story to the group and discuss the purpose and importance of getting worries out and sharing them with an adult they can trust. The message conveyed is that when worries are shared they seem less fearsome.
- Worry dolls
  Have the group of children create a worry doll from pipe cleaners and wool. Each group member is welcome to participate in naming their worry doll and giving it at least two worries. Each night the child can give one of its own worries to the doll.

This activity focuses on assisting children with their worries and encourages them to share their worries. This activity can also help if a child is having nightmares.
- Helping hand (increasing the child's support network)
  Ask each child to draw around their hand. At the point of every finger and thumb ask the group who they can think of to help them when they have a problem and need to talk to an adult who they can trust; for example, this could be a teacher, Childline, a play worker or grandparent. The facilitator can offer the group local support networks the children can use for advice and support.
- 'Nifflenoo called Nevermind' written by Margot Sunderland (a story for children who bottle up their feelings)
  Read the story and follow up with discussion about having different feelings. Ask the children to lie down on large pieces of card and get the group to draw around each other. On the picture of themselves, get the group to draw in facial features and any feelings they have been bottling up for a while, using different colours, textures and materials.
- Masks (what we show people on the outside/inside)
  Focus on the exploration of hidden feelings – how the child perceives themselves and how they wish to be perceived. Masks encourage an exploration of emotional literacy and the ability to self-express in a visual way and they act as conversation starters.

  Each activity ends with 'feel good' cards. This allows the children to explore how they feel about other people and how other people might feel about them. It can build confidence and self-esteem. For example, with a 'friendly' card – 'I have given you this card because you smiled at me when I came into the group which made me feel welcome'.

  These practical activities can help the play specialist get to know the children with whom they are working. Children who can identify and share their anxieties learn that they are not alone in their experiences and can therefore feel less isolated.

One to one play as a therapeutic intervention for children affected by domestic violence

There are three main principles of one to one play intervention; first, play is the child's medium where they feel comfortable, empowered and valued. Second, play can be, but is not always, a reflection of the child's inner world. And, third, the child has an inner drive toward play, which inherently has the potential to enhance emotional health and development across domains.

The play specialist provides an environment that allows children to feel in control of their play (Howard and McInnes, 2013). However, it is important during play sessions for children who have experienced domestic violence that the freedom to have choice and control is carefully balanced with the child's need to feel emotionally and physically safe. The play specialist can do this by setting clear limits and boundaries, similar to those adopted by play therapists. For example, the child is not permitted to:

- injure themselves or others
- damage property
- stay beyond their time
- remove toys from the playroom or play circle.

When working with children who have been exposed to domestic violence, there are two locations where play is likely to take place – a dedicated playroom or a play circle. The playroom is a permanent room used by the play specialist within the organisation to provide play sessions. The play circle is created using a mobile play kit taken along by the play specialist to use in a dedicated room within a school, nursery, family centre or community room. The play equipment in the mobile kit is presented in a circle that offers a safe consistent place for the child to play. In both settings, it is important to provide consistency; for example, if the play session is with the mobile play kit, the sessions will always take place in the same location. If the child is living in refuge accommodation, where playrooms are often communal areas, a designated room with dedicated equipment specifically for therapeutic play might be provided. The most important aim is to provide a safe environment for the child. By creating this safe environment, the play specialist can become a trusted co-player and the child can gain maximum therapeutic benefit from their play.

To meet the play needs of children at different development levels, providing resources which enable embodied play, projective play and role play is important (Jennings, 1999). Play materials which are open-ended facilitate choice and individuality; however, some materials, particularly those related to home life, are particularly important for children who have been exposed to domestic violence. The play kit used by practitioners in my team includes:

- animals (farm, zoo, wild, dinosaurs …)
- vehicles (cars, diggers, trains, lorries, boats, planes …)
- small world figures
- tea set
- finger puppets with different characters

- play dough, clay
- small bricks (Lego, blocks)
- doll's house furniture
- sand and water
- fabrics (silk, wool, scarfs with different textures ...)
- musical instruments
- pots and pans
- baby with feeding bottle, dummies, blanket
- tool set
- natural materials (shells, pebbles, driftwood, twigs, pebbles, stones ...).

Piaget (1962) described several types of play including compensatory play – a child who witnesses or experiences something unpleasant, such as domestic violence, may play this out this in order to disassociate the unpleasant act from its context (Smith-Stover *et al.* 2006). When children are affected by domestic abuse, the emphasis of the support offered is often not only hearing the 'voice of the child' but also empowering children to overcome their difficulties. McGee (2000) found that children wanted to talk about the violence but were frightened to do so. Children stated that they did not want to tell teachers or school counsellors because doing so might make it worse. They also said that they needed help in describing what they had witnessed and furthermore they needed to have accessible places in which to talk about it (Rivett, Howarth and Harold, 2006; McGee, 2000; Thatcher 2012).

Putting the control and choice back in the hands of the child is a fundamental principle of therapeutic play (Howard and McInnes, 2013). Using a non-directive approach which combines the principles of both playwork and play therapy can be particularly beneficial to a child affected by domestic violence, as it can restore a sense of control and offer feelings of empowerment otherwise unattainable in the child's life. By making their own toy selections and deciding what to play and how others are involved, children can express themselves freely (Axline, 1969; Carroll, 1998). The child can resolve difficulties through play in their own way and in their own time (Carroll, 2002).

Case study – Katie (aged 8)

Social services referred Katie to me for therapeutic play sessions due to exposure to domestic violence. Katie appeared to be withdrawn, tired and was often upset. She did not want to play with her peers and would often say she was feeling unwell during playtime and lunch so she was able to stay with her teacher or the dinner lady. The class teacher had difficulty at the end of the day with Katie's behaviour, as she never wanted to go home from school. The family had a complex background of domestic abuse, drug and alcohol misuse. Her mum had had numerous abusive partners and Katie did not have any contact with her father. Mum also had mental health problems. Support was put in place for mum within the home. Katie started attending therapeutic play sessions. She would be quiet whilst we walked to the playroom; however, as soon as she entered the 'safe' circle Katie immediately responded and appeared empowered by having control over what we played. Katie would often tell me what to do, dress me up and ask me to sing and dance. She would often laugh at the fact that I was doing what she asked, as if testing whether the play was really 'hers'. At the start of the process, Katie directed me to act out what she wanted whilst she stood on the edge of the circle. She would shout demands and on a few occasions, I had to remind Katie gently of the limits and boundaries about safety. Over the course of the play sessions, however, Katie became less overtly directive and started to engage with the toys; she took on a more playful role. I became the observer within the play circle and Katie would use the puppets and animals to play out what she needed. School reported a difference in Katie, especially on days when she was receiving therapeutic play intervention. After the session, Katie would appear more relaxed in class, energised, happy and more confident.

This case study shows Katie needed to have some power and control back in her life. Katie needed to be listened to and the therapeutic play intervention gave her the freedom to use the space as she wanted and needed. When a child is directing their own play, they have a sense of control; the child decides the rules and boundaries and the play moves with the child's interest and thought (Carroll, 2002). As the play specialist, I listened and accepted Katie's play without judging or correcting. The message given to Katie was, 'I am here, I hear you, I understand and I care' (Landreth, 2002). For the neglected child with attachment difficulties this process can help to restore faith in the nature of human relationships.

Case study – Matthew (aged 6)

Matthew and his family (Mum; John, half-brother aged 8; Anthony, brother aged 9 months) moved into a women's aid refuge, fleeing dangerous levels of domestic violence from Matthew's father. The family had moved out of area and Matthew had to start a new school. Matthew was sometimes violent towards his mum, siblings and other children in school. Refuge staff reported that Matthew's behaviour could be challenging; he would damage toys in the playroom, threaten staff and other women living in refuge. Refuge staff also reported Matthew would state 'I'm like my dad' when reprimanded for his behaviour; they described Matthew as a confused and angry child. Staff from his new school stated that he would go up to other children and hit them for no reason and was difficult to settle in the classroom. Matthew would be agitated and needed to be 'kept busy' within the classroom and refuge environment.

Matthew found being in the play circle difficult; he would often jump in and out of the circle, his play was chaotic at first, picking up different toys frenetically, not wanting to be looked at or for me to see what he was doing. Matthew would make threats – 'I'm going to smash your face with this car' – and I had to keep restating our play circle rules quite frequently. However, in time, Matthew's play became more settled; he stopped making threats and stayed for longer periods in the play circle. Matthew seemed to learn to trust in the consistency of the environment and started to play, although he continued to want to keep his play a secret, often going to the opposite side of the circle, with his back to me. Matthew was drawn to the animals. He explored how the cows were similar, but different, and I once noticed him whispering to the cow, 'You look similar to your brother, but you are different'. Matthew explored this play theme for a few sessions using different animals each week. He would give each animal a characteristic; for example, 'this cow was also angry' and 'everyone liked this cow' as 'he was kind'. Matthew played with the angry cow quite often. The cow didn't want to be angry and wanted to have other friends. Matthew acted out violent play and would take on a protective role; he would stop the violence in the play and send the 'baddy' to prison. However, the 'baddy' would always escape and find them.

Matthew had difficulty adapting to the refuge environment and starting a new school. It was clear that Matthew, at the beginning of our session, did not feel 'safe' and found being in the play space difficult. Control during his play gave Matthew the time and opportunity to develop his play skills and explore some of the difficulties he was having in his life. He explored the differences between himself and his half brother. Matthew had witnessed a lot of the domestic abuse within the home and perhaps because he looked like his father, he felt that he was a similar person. My role in Matthew's play sessions was simply to be present, maintaining the safe space where his play could evolve and develop. Through Matthew's play I was also able to gain a better understanding of how he was feeling about his experiences and he was referred for further support.

Conclusion

Domestic violence can have a detrimental impact on child witnesses as well as victims, and whilst support for victims is well established, increased support services recognising the needs of children are much needed. Children may experience a wide range of behavioural, physical and psychological effects, which may be short and/or long term.

Our understanding of how exposure to domestic violence can impact on children's development is increasing; however, it is questionable whether there are enough resources available to meet demand, particularly in relation to important early interventions which have the potential to reduce the demand for remedial, specialist services. Women's Aid and other statutory and voluntary groups are already struggling to meet the needs of the families and children with whom they work and have long waiting lists.

When a child lives in an unsafe home environment, whether this is due to abuse or neglect, they may have had fewer opportunities for play or restricted play experiences. In an environment with domestic violence, where children may receive less parental attention or parental care which lacks consistency, the development of skills and experiences of appropriate social interaction could be restricted (Copper and Sutton, 1999). This may impact on the development of play and subsequently other developmental domains.

Play can be far from fun; it can be irrational and chaotic, with a darkness that often appears to contrast with what we believe play ought to be (O'Conner, 2000). Play is inherently therapeutic, helping troubled children cope with their distress and acting as a means of communication between the child and the adult co-player. Cattanach (2003) states that play is the place where children first recognise the separateness of what is 'me' and 'not me', and begin to develop a relationship with the world beyond the self. It is the child's way of making contact with their environment.

Having the space and time to play within a safe environment is inherently therapeutic, acting at a preventative level with the aim of reducing further need for specialist support services. Early intervention with a therapeutic play specialist also facilitates referral to specialist support services as soon as possible, whenever necessary.

Key points

1. Within the UK it is estimated 750,000 children are exposed to domestic abuse each year. In 90 per cent of domestic violence incidents a child is present or in the adjacent room.
2. Children who witness abuse and live in a violent environment are at risk of serious behavioural and other psychological problems.

3. Play is an important and powerful natural resource for children affected by domestic violence:

- Early intervention through therapeutic play sessions supports the development of children's play skills and offers inherent healing potential. As such it can prevent the manifestation of behavioural or psychological problems.
- Early play intervention facilitates our understanding of children's experiences and feelings, enabling referral for further support at the earliest possible point at a remedial level.

4. Non-directive play techniques offer control to children who, when they have been exposed to domestic violence, may feel that much of their environment is chaotic and otherwise out of their control.

References

10,000 Safer Lives Project. (2012). Welsh Government. Available online at http://wales.gov.uk/topics/improvingservices/pslg/nwp/effectservices/10ksaferlivesreport/?lang=en (accessed 3 April 2013).

Axline, V. (1969). *Play Therapy*. United Kingdom: Ballentine Books.

Bandura, A. (1977). *Social Learning Theory*. Englewood Cliffs, NJ: Prentice Hall.

Brandon, M., Sidebotham, P., Bailey, S., Belderson, P., Hawley, P., Ellis, C. and Megson, M. (2012). *New Learning from Serious Case Reviews: A two year report for 2009–2011*. London: Department for Education.

Bunting, L. (2011). *The Prevalence of Infant Abuse and Maltreatment Related Deaths in the UK: A research briefing*. London: National Society for the Prevention of Cruelty to Children.

Carroll, J. (1998). *Introduction to Therapeutic Play*. Oxford: Blackwell Scientific.

Carroll, J. (2002). Play therapy: the children's views. *Child and Family Social Work*, 7 (3), pp. 177–187.

Cattanach, A. (2003). *Play Therapy with Abused Children*. London: Jessica Kingsley Publishers.

Cawson, P. (2002). *Child Maltreatment in the Family: The experience of a national sample of young people*. London: National Society for the Prevention of Cruelty to Children.

Chiodo, D., Leschied, A. W., Whitehead, P. C. and Hurley, D. (2008). Child welfare practice and policy related to the impact of children experiencing physical victimization and domestic violence. *Children and Youth Services Review*, 30 (4), pp. 564–574.

Cleaver, H., Nicholson, D., Tarr, S. and Cleaver, D. (2007). *Child Protection, Domestic Violence and Parental Substance Misuse.* London: Jessica Kingsley Publishers.
Copper, R. and Sutton, K. (1999). The effects of child abuse on preschool children's play. *Australian Journal of Early Childhood*, 24 (2), pp. 10–54.
Department of Health. (2002). *Women's Mental Health: Into the mainstream, strategic development of mental health care for women.* London: Crown.
Dowd, N., Singer, D. G. and Wilson, R. F. (2006). *Handbook of Children, culture and violence.* London: Sage Publications.
Drotar, D., Flannery, D., Day, E., Friedman, S., Creeden, R., Gartland, H., McDavid, L., Tame, C. and McTaggart, M. J. (2003). Identifying and responding to the mental health service needs of children who have experienced violence: a community-based approach. *Clinical Child Psychology and Psychiatry*, 8 (2), pp. 187–203.
Erikson, E. (1965). *Children and Society.* Harmondsworth: Penguin.
Freud, S. (1961). *Beyond the Pleasure Principle.* New York: Norton.
Glaser, D. (2000). Child abuse and neglect and the brain – a review. *Journal of Child Psychology and Psychiatry and Allied Disciplines*, 41 (1), pp. 97–116.
Holden, G. W. and Ritchie, K. L. (1991). Linking extreme marital discord, child rearing and child behaviour problems: evidence from battered women. *Child Development*, 62 (2), pp. 311–327.
Home Office (2013). *New Government Domestic Violence and Abuse Definition.* Available online at www.gov.uk/government/publications/new-government-domestic-violence-and-abuse-definition (accessed 20 July 2013).
Howard, J. (2009). Play, learning and development in early years. In T. Maynard and N. Thomas (eds), *An Introduction to Early Childhood Studies.* London: Sage.
Howard, J. and McInnes, K. (2013). *The Essence of Play: A practice companion for professionals working with children and young people.* Oxford: Routledge.
Huth-Bocks, A. C., Levendosky, A. A. and Semel, M. A. (2001). The direct and indirect effects of domestic violence on young children's intellectual functioning. *Journal of Family Violence*, 16 (3), pp. 269–290.
Jennings, S. (1999). *Introduction to Developmental Play Therapy: Playing and Health.* London: Jessica Kingsley.
Landreth, G. L. (2002). *Play Therapy: The Art of the Relationship.* UK: Brunner-Routledge.
Levy, A. (2008). The therapeutic action of play in the psychodynamic treatment of children: a critical analysis. *Clinical Social Work Journal*, 36 (3), pp. 281–291.
McGee, C. (2000). *Childhood Experiences of Domestic Violence.* London: Jessica Kingsley.
Moyles, J. (2005). *Excellence of Play.* Maidenhead: Open University Press.
NSPCC. (2011). *Child Abuse and Neglect in the UK Today.* London: NSPCC. Available online at www.nspcc.org.uk/Inform/research/findings/child_abuse_neglect_research_wda84173.html (accessed 13 May 2013).
O'Conner, J. O. (2000). *The Play Therapy Primer.* John Wiley and Sons: New York.

Peled, E. and Davis, D. (1995). *Groupwork with children of battered women: A practitioner's manual.* Thousand Oaks, CA: Sage Publications.

Piaget, J. (1962). *Play dreams and imitations in childhood.* New York: W. W. Norton

Rivett, M. J., Howarth, E. and Harold, G. (2006). 'Watching from the stairs': towards an evidence-based practice in work with child witnesses of domestic violence. *Clinical Child Psychology and Psychiatry*, 11 (1), pp. 103–125.

Shepard, M. and Raschick, M. (1999). How child welfare workers assess and intervene around issues of domestic violence. *Child Maltreatment*, 4 (2), pp. 148–156.

Smith-Stover, C., Van-Horn, P. and Lieberman, A. F. (2006). Parental representations in the play of preschool aged witness of marital violence. *Journal of Family Violence*, 21 (5), 417–424.

Spilbury, J. C., Belliston, L., Drotar, D., Drinkard, A., Kretschmar, J., Creeden, R., Flannery, D. and Friedman, S. (2007). Clinically significant trauma symptom and behavioural problems in a community-based sample of children exposed to domestic violence. *Journal of Family Violence*, 22 (8), pp. 487–499.

Stone, B. (1998). Child neglect: practitioners' perspectives. *Child Abuse Review*, 7 (2), pp. 87–96.

Stover, C. S. (2005). Domestic violence research: what have we learned and where do we go from here? *Journal of Interpersonal Violence*, 20 (4), pp. 448–454.

Thatcher, C. (2012). *'You've Given Us a Voice, Now Listen', Children and Young People's Research Project.* Wales: Welsh Women's Aid.

Thoburn, J., Wilding, J. and Watson, J. (2000). *Family Support in Cases of Emotional Maltreatment and Neglect.* London: The Stationery Office.

Tsao, L. (2002). How much do we know about the importance of play in child development. *Childhood Education*, 78 (4), pp. 230–242.

Vygotsky, L. S. (1967). Play and its role in the mental development of the child. *Soviet Psychology*, 5 (3), pp. 6–18.

Walby, S. (2009). *The Cost of Domestic Violence Update.* UK: Lancaster University.

Welsh Assembly Government (2012). Consultation on legislation to end violence against women and domestic abuse (Wales). Available online at http://wales.gov.uk/consultations/housingcommunity/vawwhitepaper/?lang=en (accessed 3 April 2013).

Ybarra, G. J., Wilkens, S. L. and Lieberman, A. F. (2007). The influence of domestic violence on preschooler behaviour and functioning. *Journal of Family Violence*, 22 (1), pp. 33–42.

11 Using play therapeutically with groups

5

Applying an Embodiment-Projection-Role framework in groupwork with children

Sue Jennings

There are two interweaving developmental paradigms, Neuro-Dramatic-Play (NDP) (Jennings, 2011a), and Embodiment-Projection-Role (EPR) (Jennings, 1990), which form the core of creative groupwork with children. Rather like the chains of DNA, NDP and EPR create curls and swirls of how we think about the creative play process and how we apply it with groups (and individuals). Above all, the emphasis is on play and its essential contribution to the health of children (Bruner *et al.* 1985; Sutton-Smith, 2001).

This chapter looks at the underlying theory and the group application of both NDP and EPR and how they can be facilitated for social and emotional growth, particularly with children who struggle with their communication and behaviour. It is likely that many of these children will have attachment difficulties, but this chapter is not about clinical therapy – it is about the facilitation of creative and therapeutic groupwork to enhance personal and social strengths.

NDP and EPR are 'value free'; they do not rely on a particular school of psychological theory or model of therapy and they can be integrated into any psychological model or therapeutic or educational practice. Developments in Positive Psychology (Seligman, 2002) have continued to influence NDP and EPR, particularly in emphasising children's strengths rather than their deficits.

Description of NDP and EPR

Neuro-Dramatic-Play is the earliest embodied development that commences six months before birth and continues until six months after birth. It is characterised by 'sensory, rhythmic and dramatic play' and influences the growth of healthy attachments (Jennings, 2011a). It is an expansion of the Embodiment stage that commences at birth and continues to 13 months, the most significant growth period for children. The body houses physical well-being, sensory play and creative expression. There is the greatest impact on the brain–body connection during these months.

Embodiment-Projection-Role (EPR) is a developmental paradigm that uniquely follows the progression of dramatic play from birth to seven years. Based on extended observations with babies, young children and pregnant women, it provides a parallel progression alongside other developmental processes such as physical, cognitive, emotional and social.

NDP and EPR chart the 'dramatic development' of children, which is the basis of the child being able to enter the world of imagination and symbolism, the world of ritualistic and dramatic play, and drama. The early attachment between mother and infant has a strong dramatic component through playfulness and 'role-reversal'. Even in pregnancy the mother is forming a dramatic relationship with her unborn child.

Competence in NDP and EPR are essential for a child's maturation as they:

- create the core of attachment between mother and infant
- form a basis for the growth of identity and independence
- establish the 'dramatised body' i.e. the body which can create
- strengthen and further develop the imagination
- contribute to a child's resilience through 'ritual and risk'(Jennings, 1998)
- enable a child to move appropriately from 'everyday reality' to 'dramatic reality' and back again (Jennings 1990)
- facilitate problem solving and conflict resolution
- provide role play and dramatic play which in turn create flexibility
- give a child the experience and skills to be part of the social world.

Embodiment-Projection-Role provide the markers of life changes that are ritualised through playing and drama from one stage to the next.

Embodiment including NDP

During the Embodiment (E) stage we can see how the child's early experiences are physicalised and are mainly expressed through bodily movement and the senses. The child develops security and trust (Erikson, 1965, 1995), through the early physical attachment of NDP: sensory, rhythmic and dramatic playfulness, that then flow into a relaxed, attuned relationship. Through these embodied experiences, the infant is establishing interactive communication through touch and sound, and rhythmic and ritualistic repetition.

These body-focussed activities are essential for the development of the 'body-self': we cannot have a body image until we have a body-self

(Jennings, 1998). The child needs to be able to 'live' in his or her body, which grows from being a secure part of the mother's body. The progression is from being inside the mother, to being closely attached to the mother, and then gradually becoming independent, with the opportunity to resume physical contact, when desired or when fearful. This will establish the infant's security to feel confident about moving in space. This progression can also be described as the three circles of attachment: the circle within the womb; the circle in mother's arms; the symbolic circle when the mother 'holds' the infant in her consciousness and is attuned to changes in moods and needs.

Most of our early physical and bodily experience comes through our proximity to others, usually our mothers or carers (I shall continue to use the word mother in a generic sense of the person who cares for us). We are cradled and rocked as we co-operate with rhythmic rocking and singing. Babies respond and mothers respond again; there is a collaborative approach to physical expression. Already the movement takes on some ritual/risk qualities: on the one hand we have ritualised rocking movement and, on the other hand, bounce up and down with glee. Ritual and risk are the dual components of early physical play, where infants feel safely held and contained on the one hand, but contrastingly enjoy the thrill of the 'danger' (Jennings, 1998). I learn about my own body by being bodily engaged with another, thus I am 'mimetically engaged' (see Wilshire, 1982, Chapters 3 and 4).

The body is the *primary means of learning* (Jennings, 1990) and all other learning is secondary to that first learned through the body. Therefore, children with body trauma need extended *physical play* in order to re-build a healthy and confident body. A child's embodiment development can be distorted through the following (Jennings, 1999):

- Being 'over-held' – the child who is over protected, over dependent; there is a perpetual fused state and a blurring of body-boundaries. The child is always physically 'with' the mother and has never separated or been 'against' her, (Sherborne, 2001).
- Being 'under-held' – the child who is left for long periods of time in isolation; develops anxiety rather than autonomy, is mistrustful and often confused about body and spatial boundaries.
- Being violated through physical or sexual abuse – the child's bodily boundaries are invaded with resultant trauma and confusion; there is often fear and anxiety and either an avoidance of physical contact or inappropriate physical rage or un-boundaried touch.

Many therapists find it difficult to consider using Embodiment in their work because of traumatic experiences in the child's or therapist's past, or with the ever-present fear of misunderstood touch and possible litigation. Parents need to know that touch is involved in creative workshops.

Working in groups and doing group movement is very good for social development. Not all movement has to involve touch and there are many healing movement games for children and practitioners to do together, including working with various 'props' such as hoops, string, or silk scarves (the scarf establishes a contact with the children – this is also especially useful when working with children on the autistic spectrum).

Useful Neuro-Dramatic-Play and Embodiment Techniques *(see Jennings 1995, 1999, 2010a, 2011a, 2011b, 2013a, 2013b; Sherborne, 2001)*

- appropriate massage, on the upper back and shoulders, or hands
- singing games which name hands, feet, eyes, nose and so on
- clapping songs with words and movements
- drum rhythms and echoes
- gross body movement involving the whole body
- rocking and chanting in pairs: 'Row, Row, Row the Boat'
- fine body movement with different body parts
- blowing bubbles and catching them
- sensory movement involving textures, sound, taste, smell and sight
- rhythmic movement and dance
- movement games such as 'Simon says...'
- rough and tumble play
- messy play with finger paints, sand and water
- creative ideas of moving as monsters, aliens, mice
- stories with sounds and movement.

Transition one
Around 12–14 months we can observe the time of transition from the body to the world 'out there' – the world of projection and objects that are separate from the personal body. As Winnicott (1974) has suggested, the first attachment to an object – often soft and cuddly such as a blanket or shawl – marks the transition to other objects, just as the attachment to the mother will lead to healthy attachments to other people.

However the object itself is not just a ritual symbol, representing the absent mother, it is also a creative object that can turn into many things and be played with. It almost always has a name and it has to stay the same (woe-betide whoever puts the transitional object (TO) in the washing machine), but it also becomes personified and is talked to. It can be a hiding place or a mask – the TO is a prime example of both flexibility and ritual and risk.

Projection

During the Projective stage (13 months to 3 years), the child is responding to the world beyond the body and to things outside the body. The child's responses may well be physical – for example, when a child plays with finger paint – but the important point is that the paint is a substance outside the body boundaries. Just as the transitional object moves the child from the embodiment to the projective stage, messy play starts as sensory and embodied play to a more ordered and controlled projective activity.

As the Projective (P) stage develops, children not only relate to different objects and substances, they also place them together in shapes and constellations. There is such a delight in building with bricks and then knocking them down again! There is a large range of art activities, painting, sticking, and colouring. Children are discovering their own emerging order. Soon we see an increasing use of stories through play with objects such as the dolls' house or small toys.

As children develop more and more into the P stage we notice them moving from exploratory play where things are tasted and tested, to more patterned and organised play with objects, and then to more dramatized play with stories. Although it has these variations, it is still projective play – that is, it is play *beyond* the body, and objects take on roles and meanings. Without confusing the issue, we could even say that the P stage has EPR stages within it as described below. However, it is clear on closer examination that all the activities are projective ones:

- E – when the child is sensorily exploring media such as finger paint and water play.
- P – 'pure' projection when bricks are built, patterns are made, pictures are crayoned, collages are created.
- R – when stories are told with the dolls' house or scenes are made with animals (sculpting).

Useful projective techniques (see Astell-Burt, 2001; Cattanach, 1994; Jennings, 2004, 2011b, 2013a, 2013b; Jennings and Minde, 1993; Smith, 2012)

Play with:

- natural media: pebbles, bark, twigs, leaves
- junk materials from scrap shops and re-cycling
- substance: sand, water, finger paint, clay, play dough

- pictures: crayons, paints, drawing, collage with varied media
- bricks and counters: patterns, constructions, 'all fall down'
- small world toys: sand tray stories, sculpts
- scenes: dolls' house, and also puppet-making.

Children can be encouraged to create in different media, and workers may create at the same time so the child does not feel scrutinised. The children can co-create an artistic construction or a den or a house, thus building a shared endeavour. The children lead the creative partnership.

Transition two
We can observe towards the end of the P stage that a child's play is becoming more and more 'dramatised' with stories and scenes being enacted from newly created stories, or stories that already exist. Children are developing their own narrative structures, stories that have a beginning, middle and an end. They are also increasing their capacity for 'free-play', what adults would term improvisation, where you start with a topic or an object and see where it goes. We could also refer to this process as 'stream of consciousness', which may well feed into a later narrative structure, but is invaluable as a life skill.

During this transition we can observe children become their own directors and the directors of others as they organise 'events' and create plays in which they both perform and direct. They often acquire symbols of authority such as sticks, magic batons or special uniforms or costumes. They are able to exist separately with their creativity as well as being part of a pair or small group. Eventually the child starts to take on the roles, sometimes several in a scene, and we can observe the emergence of the Role stage. There is a development of 'what is right' for a scene or a role – such as, 'mummies don't do that' or 'monsters walk like this'. Not only are roles enacted but also scenes are directed, and there is an increasing awareness of design and staging.

Role

It is gradually being accepted that people learn about themselves and others by playing a role of someone else (Jennings, 1990, 2011a, 2011b, 2013a, 2013b; Landy, 1993; Wilshire, 1982; Smilanksy, 1968; Mead, 1934).

Dramatic play, or the Role (R) stage, is the culmination of the primary NDP/EPR stages and is usually complete by about the age of seven years. We can see a difference in the 'drama' of children at this age from the 'dramatic play' of the years before. The Role stage involves children taking on roles in stories from texts or through improvisation, and involving the facilitator and other things in the role – chairs draped with material, large toys and so on, can all take on roles within the scene. Children may make and wear masks, and masks should be a part of the play therapists' equipment.

It is crucial that the character and the scene, and indeed the space, are 'de-roled' (Jennings 1990) before the session is ended. The child needs to be very clear what belongs to the dramatic reality of the story or the play, and what belongs to the everyday reality of their world. 'Anything is possible within the drama, and the dramatic play gives permission to do things, that in everyday life would not be either permissible or wholesome' (Jennings, 2002, p. 3), and Berg (1998) suggests that '[b]y taking the part of a role-play you can become the person you are acting' (p. 3).

It is important that the children have the opportunity to play 'distanced' roles – that is, those that are in stories and plays. In doing so, the child is likely to come nearer to their own experience than if they enact their specific, immediate situation. This is the paradox of drama – 'that I come closer by being more distanced' (Jennings, 1998, p. 116). This also is the hardest thing for therapeutic workers to handle, because we all want to know 'what is going on'. Maybe we have to learn to bear 'not knowing', 'to stay with the chaos and allow the meaning to emerge' (Jennings, 1987, p. 2).

Useful role and story techniques (see Jennings, 1999, 2010a, 2011a, 2011b, 2013a, 2013b; McFarlane, 2005; Slade, 1954; Spolin, 1986; Stagnitti and Cooper, 2009)

- use simple roles with single feelings: the angry person, the sad person and maybe draw the faces of the people
- use large boxes and pieces of cloth to enable children to develop their own ideas
- create animal characters that interact
- use favourite stories to enact together
- use the dressing up box to allow a dramatised story to emerge
- use a mask as a starting point for a story
- use ideas that have been generated through projective play.

Horley (1998) has done extensive research using the EPR method in order to identify children who are 'non-players'. She suggests that dramatic play is:

> a situation where role playing becomes more complex and includes dressing up, developing dialogue and creating environments within which to play different roles.
>
> (p. 3)

It is as if the children have fully integrated Embodiment, Projection and Role as they create plays with movement, sounds, costumes, props and various characters. Usually the three stages of E and P and R are completed by the age of seven years. However it does not stop there. People continue to visit these stages in pre-teen and teenage development, not necessarily always in the EPR sequence. Nevertheless they are experimented with, tried and tested as identity continues to develop. Finally we make choices as adults based on the stage that we have dominance in, and usually take up jobs and hobbies that have either an E or P or R focus. Conflict or distress can ensue if we make a life choice that is not based on our own personality but comes from the pressure and expectations of others.

Therapeutic groupwork in practice

It would be easy to assume that now we have a rationale, a progression and a range of techniques, we just go and activate the process. However we need to reflect on the actual process of planning and facilitating groupwork with children. It is not a question of designing a syllabus; rather it is providing the right context and environment to encourage creativity and spontaneity. What is needed for children to flourish?

Children need a secure structure with 'signposts' in order for their own creativity to develop as individuals and in collaboration with others. Basic social skills with pairs, small and large groups, can be learned and practised through creative groupwork. For example, planning a journey through the magic forest needs organisation, decision-making, management, role skills, observation, alertness.... This is done by the children (or young people) themselves within a structure provided by the group facilitator (play therapist or other appropriately qualified professional).

The philosophy behind this work is the empowering of children and young people, which means allowing them to develop at their own pace and in their own rhythm. In ideal circumstances, children regulate themselves in developmental sequences without having to be directed. Children and young people with developmental delay, or developmental trauma, will often need to catch up through the NDP/EPR stages. Part of the task of the group facilitator is to have available materials that are both age and stage appropriate. For example, teenagers may well feel that finger painting is childish, but they can get very messy if they model with clay, or squirt paint directly from bottles! They may initially reject a fairy tale, but will usually know the characters in 'Big Bang Theory' (Jennings, 2013a). These characters are geeks who struggle with their social skills, which make them ideal as roles for young people to explore. Teenagers will shy away from anything that might make them look foolish or that may seem childish. It is important to have a large portfolio of materials that can be adapted for many situations, within the EPR framework (Jennings, 2004). Such a portfolio includes:

- a wide range of warm-up activities and drama games
- ideas for physical activities including sensory and messy play
- examples of rhythmic play and the use of drumming and clapping
- materials for diverse art work including worksheets, collage ideas, and art supplies
- stories: myths and fairy tales; therapeutic stories; creative visualisation ideas; poems and rap songs (Jennings 2005)
- drama ideas and themes: from stories, from everyday life, from TV (Swale, 2009; Jennings, 2013a).

Resources need to be available together with an appropriate space, where children can move around, sit comfortably on the floor, use messy play, and make noise!

Suggested equipment includes recycled materials (as much as possible): boxes large and small, coloured wrappers, wool and string, newspapers and magazines, scraps of fabric; bubbles; crayons, paints and brushes; glue, scissors, stapler; flour and water or clay or Plasticine; sticks for puppet making (Jennings, 2006); simple dressing-up clothes (a wide variety of hats and caps, scarves, cloaks, shawls, belts and large pieces of fabric).

Facilitation skills for creative groupwork

Pre-planning

Participants: Consider where participants will come from. Are they to be referred or can parents book directly? Written consent is needed if the children, or their artwork, are to be photographed (if that is part of the plan).
Group size: If one person is facilitating there may be 3–8 children; if two people are co-facilitating there could be more. However, group size will vary depending on age (the younger the children the smaller the group), whether the children are typically developing and attending for fun and creative expression (rather than as an intervention to address difficulties) and also on the target group and their concentration, attention span, particular difficulties, and any developmental delay. Mixed gender groups are fine up to the age of seven, thereafter work with just boys or just girls is generally best.

Central theme, aims and objectives: Activities throughout each programme and each session are linked to a central theme that serves as a structure for varied and linked activities, in keeping with the programme's aims and objectives. It is important to choose a theme that will engage the participants and select and apply activities in an age and stage appropriate sequence. There should be a clear rationale for the choice of each activity.

NDP/EPR groupwork structure

- A series of sessions may focus on basic sensory, rhythmic and dramatic play, which provides the groundwork for establishing healthy attachments through creative playing.
- A single session may include the EPR sequence (see sample sessions below).
- A series of sessions may progress through the EPR sequence: first sessions focusing on Embodiment; middle sessions on Projection; final session on Role.
- Progression from one stage to the next happens when a group is ready to move on. Some groups may stay at the Embodiment stage until they build enough confidence and grounding to move on. Others may not move on at all, especially if they are not developmentally ready for Projection and/or Role play.

Facilitating the sessions

Instructions: Ground rules need to be precise and clear, and times for starting and ending the sessions.
Contract: An agreement needs to be made with every group that includes basic ground rules: for example, no one gets hurt either physically or through words; equipment is not broken or destroyed; everyone's work is respected, including art work or ideas that people contribute; everyone listens to what others have to say.
Structure: Every session has a clear beginning, middle and ending (leading to closure): the beginning is the warm-up(s), introduction of a story or theme; the middle is the main focus of the action; the end is the cool-down, reflection, sharing and closure. One thing needs to lead to another logically and sequentially and not be a series of unrelated exercises (see sample sessions below).
Warm-ups: Exercises and games to focus physical energy, encourage cooperation, and develop mental strategies – for example, 'Simon Says', Chain Tag', 'Fox and Lambs', 'Step in Sequence'.
Changing activities: Call out 'freeze' for everyone to stand still and listen to a new instruction, or to calm down energy if the children start to become over-excited.

Encouraging group members to contribute ideas: Phrases such as: 'Has anyone thought about... who or what lives in the forest? ... are there local stories and legends? ...what is the other side of the rainbow?'; or 'I wonder what... would happen if treasure is discovered on the beach? ...you would find under the lily-pad of the pond? ...where it would go if the school bus suddenly took a new route?' can be used to generate ideas and enrich the play.

Relationships and participation: The facilitator will be alert to the developing relationships within the group – including peer relationships and adult child relationships. Note interactions, levels of involvement and engagement and the responses of individual children to particular media and activities. Adapt plans as necessary to facilitate healthy relationships and facilitate participation. Keeping to the plan is never more important than responsive facilitation.

Evaluation: It is important that the children, however young, are encouraged to evaluate the sessions. Sheets can be created that list the activities (perhaps using images) and older children can fill one in at the end of each session, perhaps using stickers with facial expressions or marks. Larger facial expressions (perhaps drawn on paper plates) can be used with younger children (with shorter attention span and poor pencil skills) who can run to a chair holding the image that matches their experience of the particular activity that the facilitator names. Creativity is needed in facilitating evaluation as in other group activities (Jennings, 2010b).

Facilitator evaluation includes: levels of group participation; individual engagement with the theme/story as well as individual exercises; personal reflection on feelings and skills; changes that could be made another time; degree of flexibility in allowing activities to be child-led rather than directed.

Recording the sessions: Create recording sheets to suit the requirements of the particular group and commissioning agency. Consider using the following headings: names/initials that are ticked for each session; time, date, and session number; aims for session, materials, what actually happened, closing techniques; any matters for concern/actions needed; personal reflections and thoughts for the following session. Consider if the activities used were successful in achieving your aims.

Sample session 1 (can be the first of a series), based on a theme

Theme: Rainbows
Rationale: To provide a theme that is recognised by most children and that allows for imaginative responses to pictures and stories.

Resources: Multi-coloured scarves, chiffon strips; paints, crayons; worksheets; 'Rainbow Fish', 'Rainbow Fish to the Rescue' books by Marcus Pfister, (finger puppets and games also available); simple dressing-up clothes; old gloves in pale colours.
Participants: 6 boys and girls aged 5–6 years from an afterschool club.
Aims: To stimulate ideas and develop creativity and fun.

Overall session plan

Embodiment: Warm-ups can include: the 'weather map' back massage (Jennings, 2005) that ends with the rainbow; rainbow movements with arms; scarves or chiffon strips of many colours can be used for dance and movement.

Invite contributions: does anyone live on the rainbow? What might we find on the other side? Does anyone know a rainbow song? (Always accept all contributions and find ways to explore them through movement and play.)
Projection: Everyone can paint their own rainbows or make them with Plasticine or create a group painting.
Role: A rainbow story can be enacted through role-play or through a series of 'freeze-frames' – still body pictures. It can be an existing story or one that the group have created. Rainbow finger puppets can be created by cutting the fingers off gloves and colouring them in rainbow stripes.
Wind down/closure: Everyone needs to be involved in 'de-roling' and closure activities to end the session. Everyone carries their own art work or objects and places them safely in a designated place. Invite everyone to sit in a circle, close their eyes and breathe deeply three or four times; everyone then shares something they enjoyed about the session.
Evaluation sheet: List the activities with spaces for comments – comments can be made with words or drawings – or use headings with thumbs up or down signs.
NOTE: If this theme is part of a series of six sessions,

- sessions 1–2 can focus on Embodiment: include sensory play with rainbow bubbles, movement, dance, fabric and reading of the Rainbow Fish story;
- sessions 3–4 can focus on Projection: include painting rainbows, rainbow fish (what other animal might be in rainbow colours? Elmer the Elephant is a rainbow elephant);
- sessions 5–6 can move towards Role: enact a rainbow story, or make rainbow puppets and create a story.

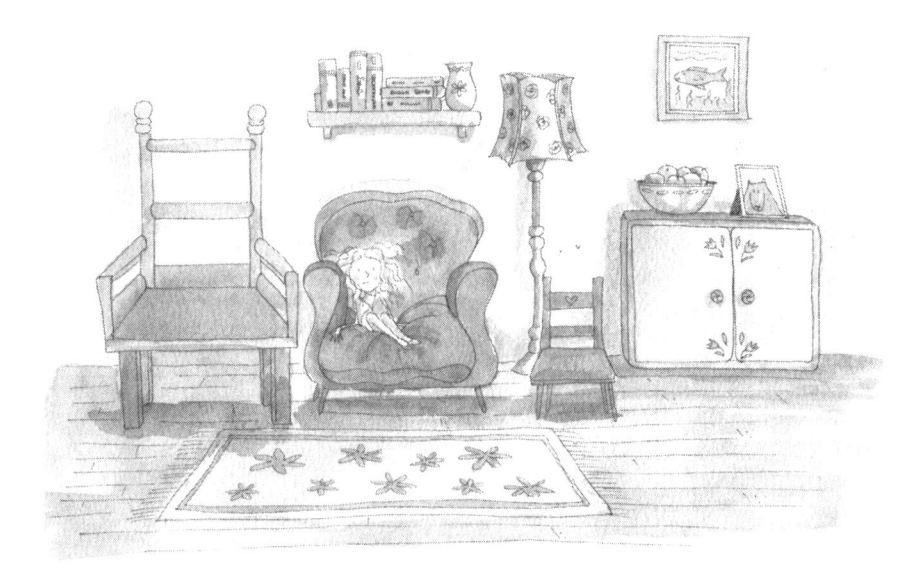

Figure 5.1 Picture of *Goldilocks and the Three Bears* by Charlie Meyer

Sample session 2 (can be part of a series), based on a story

Story: Goldilocks and the Three Bears
Rationale: To use a familiar story for creative exploration and fun.
Resources: The story, re-cycled materials (for building houses), drawing and painting materials, dressing-up clothes.
Participants: 6 children aged 4–5 years from a nursery school.
Aims: To build on an existing story to encourage individual variations and responses; to develop emotional intelligence.

Overall session plan

Warm-up: Walk as bears walking through the forest; as small children playing 'Follow My Leader'; sweet and salty things to taste (check for allergies and obtain parental permission); contrasting fabrics to explore; show different emotions felt by Goldilocks and the bears – in pairs.
Projection: Create a den or house with boxes and re-cycled materials, or paint a group picture of the forest, or colour the Three Bears pictures.
Role: Act out scenes from the story through role play or freeze frames.
Wind down/closure: Encourage everyone to run round the room as themselves and then jump three times before lying down on the floor. Invite

everyone to close their eyes and imagine all the things they have done in the session and think about what they liked and did not like; remember any fun in the session.
Evaluation: Design an appropriate evaluation sheet based on the above example (Jennings, 2010b).

NOTE: As part of a series,

- sessions 1–2 (Embodiment) can focus on exploring differences between bears' movements and children's; contrasting tastes, size, textures;
- sessions 3–4 (Projection) can build a forest house, paint bear pictures, colour pictures;
- sessions 5–6 (Role) can create and show scenes from the story, through enactment or role play.

Ideas for discussion and initiation (with this age group and older children): Ask who has heard of the story and then read it to the group. Who could move like a character in the story? What feelings are shown in the story?

There is a lot of scope for sensory exploration: the sounds, textures and smells of the forest; the taste of hot and cold porridge (or in some versions sweet and salty); the colours in the house, the texture of the fur, the clothes of the little girl.

The senses and emotions can be explored and developed by group members, and their own suggestions encouraged. Such as: How would the bears feel about someone tasting their porridge? What would the little girl feel when she woke up to see the bears? And more subtly, at the beginning, what was the girl's feeling when she went to peep inside the bear's house, after she had seen them go off for a walk.

Using the motto of 'show me' rather than 'tell me', these suggestions can be developed by the children, possibly in pair work (older children). It is important that everyone's contribution is valued and that put-down, criticism and scorn are not allowed in the ground rules.

Conclusion

Facilitating groupwork is about enabling it to happen, rather than trying to control it. So, for example, as a possible progression from all the embodiment activities suggested above, rather than telling the children to draw, a question could be asked: 'I wonder if there are other ways to tell this story?' They will almost inevitably suggest playing with small toys, drawing or puppets or drama. The small world play and art activities (drawing or painting or clay modelling) (P) would follow developmentally from the sensory play and movement (E). This is likely to lead into puppet and drama work (R). Creativity is about the children being able to explore, without fear of failure, different ideas in different media, alone and with others. Facilitators need to develop the confidence to 'allow things to emerge', within a flexible but safe structure.

Key points

1. EPR forms the core of therapeutic and developmental groupwork with children and young people.
2. It is important to recognise the EPR sequence when planning therapeutic groupwork.
3. Children of all ages can benefit from an EPR approach.

References

Astell-Burt, C. (2001). *I Am the Story: The Art of Puppetry in Education and Therapy*. London: Souvenir Press.
Berg, L. E. (1998). Developmental play stages in child identity construction; an interactionist theoretical contribution. Draft paper presented at OMEC Conference, Copenhagen 1998.
Bruner, J. L. et al. (1985). *Play: Its Role in Development and Evolution*. London: Pelican.
Cattanach, A. (1994). *Play Therapy: Where the Sky Meets the Underworld*. London: Jessica Kingsley.
Erikson, E. (1995 [1965]). *Childhood and Society*. London: Vintage.
Horley, E. (1998). Developmental assessment of dramatic play. Paper presented at OMEC Conference, Copenhagen, 1998.
Jennings, S. (1987). Developmental dramatherapy. Paper presented Tel Hai College, Israel.
Jennings, S. (1990). *Dramatherapy with Families, Groups and Individuals*. London: Jessica Kingsley.
Jennings, S. (1995). *Playing for Real*. International Play Journal, 3, pp. 132–141.
Jennings, S. (1998). *Introduction to Dramatherapy*. London: Jessica Kingsley.
Jennings, S. (1999). *Introduction to Developmental Playtherapy*. London: Jessica Kingsley.
Jennings, S. (2004). *Creative Storytelling with Children at Risk*. Bicester: Speechmark.

Jennings, S. (2005). *Creative Play with Children at Risk*. Bicester: Speechmark.
Jennings, S. (2006). *Creative Puppetry with Children and Adults*. Bicester: Speechmark.
Jennings, S. (2010a [1986]). *Creative Drama in Groupwork*. Milton Keynes: Speechmark.
Jennings, S. (2010b). Drama therapy assessment through Embodiment-Projection-Role. In D. R. Johnson, S. Pendzik and S. Snow (eds), *Assessment in Drama Therapy. Springfield*, IL: Charles C. Thomas.
Jennings, S. (2011a). *Healthy Attachments and Neuro-Dramatic-Play*. London: Jessica Kingsley.
Jennings, S. (2011b). *101 Activities for Empathy and Awareness*. Buckingham: Hinton House.
Jennings, S. (2013a). *101 Activities for Managing Challenging Behaviour*. Buckingham: Hinton House.
Jennings, S. (2013b). *101 Activities for Social and Emotional Resilience*. Buckingham: Hinton House.
Jennings, S. and Minde, A. (1993). *Art Therapy and Dramatherapy: Masks of the Soul*. London: Jessica Kingsley.
Landy, R. (1993). *Persona and Performance*. London: Jessica Kingsley.
McFarlane, P. (2005). *Dramatherapy: Developing emotional stability*. London: David Fulton.
Mead, G. H. (1934). *Mind, Self and Society*. Chicago: University of Chicago Press.
Perrow, S. (2012). *Therapeutic Storytelling: 101 Healing Stories for Children*. Stroud: Hawthorn Press.
Pfister, M. (2007). *The Rainbow Fish*. New York: North South Books.
Seligman, M. (2002). *Authentic Happiness*. New York: The Free Press.
Sherborne, V. (2001). *Developmental Movement for Children*. London: Worth Publishing Ltd.
Slade, P. (1954). *Child Drama*. London: Hodder and Stoughton.
Smilansky, S. (1968). *The effects of sociodramatic play on disadvantaged preschool children*. New York: Wiley.
Smith, S. D. (2012). *Sandtray Play and Storymaking*. London: Jessica Kingsley.
Spolin, V. (1986). *Theater Games for the Classroom*. Los Angeles: North Western University Press.
Stagnitti, K. and Cooper, R. (2009). *Play as Therapy*. London: Jessica Kingsley.
Sutton-Smith, (2001). *The Ambiguity of Play*. Harvard: First Harvard University Press.
Swale, J. (2009). *Drama Games for Classroom and Workshops*. London: Nick Hern.
Wilshire, B. (1982). *Role Playing and Identity*. Indiana: Indiana University Press.
Winnicott, D. (1974). *Playing and Reality*. London: Penguin.

6

The use of puppets in therapeutic and educational settings

Siobhán Prendiville

This chapter outlines the therapeutic and educational value of puppets, detailing their various psychological and behaviour management functions. Clinical techniques, relating to choosing and using puppets, in both therapeutic and educational settings, and their theoretical underpinnings are addressed. The invaluable role of puppets in ensuring that fun and playfulness take centre stage in creative groupwork and educational settings for children is demonstrated. The use of puppets to help children gain an understanding of their world, communicate thoughts, express feelings and alter cognitive distortions is outlined. The use of puppets in targeting and improving challenging behaviours and fostering and promoting social and emotional development is discussed, as is the value of using puppets to support therapeutic storytelling. The powerful impact of using puppets in educational and therapeutic settings is illustrated using clinical vignettes.

My work as both a teacher and a play therapist has enabled me to use puppets in both therapeutic and educational settings. This work has afforded me many opportunities to witness the power puppets hold when working with children and has led me to the conclusion that puppets are, in fact, magical! In this chapter I hope to share some of this magic with you. So, what is it about puppets that make them such a powerful tool when working with children? Primarily, puppets are naturally engaging; they can look directly at a child, speak directly to a child and even shake a child's hand! When used effectively, puppets are no longer inanimate; the puppet does not merely represent a living thing, he takes on a life of his own. Puppets grab and hold children's attention, capture their imagination, and generate feelings of excitement and anticipation for people of all ages (Bentley, 2005). In addition, puppets are extremely versatile; they can be used in many different ways, by both the adult and the child (Astell-Burt, 2002). The possibilities are endless, puppets have the ability to evolve and adapt to suit the needs of a particular child or group. A puppet can be used to simply tell a story, to offer comfort to a distressed child, to model appropriate touch or breathing, and can even become a child's best friend.

Clinical applications: child's use of puppets

Many children are naturally drawn towards puppets and engage spontaneously in projective expression through them (Narcavagee, 1997). When given the opportunity, regardless of context (therapy room, or classroom environment, group work or one to one), children will play with and explore puppets in many different ways. Children's spontaneous puppet play offers a multitude of therapeutic and educational benefits.

1 *Express thoughts and feelings, gain understanding and insights*

The word puppet is linked to the word for doll: *pupa* in Latin and *pupée* in French. However, children treat and play with puppets in very different ways to dolls. 'Whereas a child or an adult will talk to dolls, they will talk through a puppet' (Jennings, 2008: 6). However, I believe that children do both – they talk to and through puppets. Children regularly project their inner thoughts and feelings onto puppets, thus facilitating affective expression (Hall *et al.* 2002, p. 520) and providing the necessary dramatic distance for some distressed children to communicate strong emotions and act out real life-experiences and situations (DeLucia-Waak, 2006, p.154). In so doing, puppets enable children to gain an understanding of their world and resolve inner conflicts. Play with puppets focuses attention away from the child and allows them to express a wide range of thoughts and feelings. Problems, fears, worries and inner conflicts are frequently voiced and demonstrated through the puppet. According to Law (2004: 16) this type of play not only helps the child to gain understanding 'but it also helps them process the problem' (as cited in DeLucia-Waack, 2006). In addition, the therapist can respond to the child's puppet play through reflection and commentary in a way that will 'reflect understanding and provide corrective emotional experiences' (Hall *et al.* 2002, p. 520). As mentioned previously, children both talk to and through puppets and the manner in which a child uses a puppet influences my therapeutic responses. When the child communicates directly through the puppet, I generally direct my therapeutic response to the puppet, not the child, thus sustaining the dramatic distance required by the child.

Jane, a five-year-old girl, utilised a large puppet named Mandy to recount bad dreams that Mandy had experienced. When this occurred I directed my responses to the puppet and effectively completed therapeutic work based on Mandy's bad dreams. At other times, a child simply talks to the puppet, sharing news, fears, and experiences. A teacher using puppets in the classroom environment overheard a child, whose mother had recently died, telling a simple sleeve puppet about his mother's death and his deep sadness. According to the teacher, and the child's father, it was the first time the child had spoken about his mother's death.

In instances like this, when a child speaks directly to a puppet, I pick it up and deliver therapeutic responses through the puppet.

2 Release fears, worries and aggression

Children worry about many things and can be prone to bottling up their feelings. Anxieties and fears may be the cause of presenting problems, such as aggressive outbursts, sibling conflicts, impulsivity, distractibility and separation anxiety. Puppets provide children with an acceptable, developmentally appropriate, means of releasing fears, aggression and frustration (Woodard and Milch, 2012). Puppet play is effective in helping children to identify and discuss their worries and fears, fostering and promoting social and emotional development. When engaging in puppet play, children have the opportunity to take on a variety of roles – the child or the parent, the bully or the bullied, the abused or the abuser. They can take on roles they fear and learn to control their anxieties. A child who is fearful going to school can select a puppet and assume the role of an angry teacher. By doing so, he can feel in control and act out his impressions of being the authority figure. In this way the child can gain control over his real fears. Play with puppets enables children to verbally and kinaesthetically express emotions, including happiness, sadness, fear, jealousy, and anger. This can help them to identify emotions in themselves and others, understand that all feelings are common and acceptable, resolve inner conflicts, and become empowered.

An eleven-year-old boy, Tom, often used puppets in this way during his play therapy sessions. Tom was adopted at ten months and was diagnosed with expressive and receptive language difficulties. He was presenting with low self-esteem and high anxiety levels, was performing below average in school and experiencing significant difficulties in peer relationships. In the therapy room Tom would direct me to gather up an audience, comprising of teddies, and sit and watch as he directed and delivered a puppet show. The main characters in his puppet show, which continued and developed over six sessions, were a young girl, a grandfather, and a number of bullies. In the beginning, his puppet show depicted a young girl being bullied in school because she had a 'slow brain'. He presented the girl's sadness, fears and worries and her desire to get a new brain. Over a number of sessions the little girl did indeed manage to get a new brain (via a magic tree), however, as time passed she was not happy with her new, 'faster thinking brain'. After much consideration, she decided to return to the magic tree and get her old brain back. The young girl's confidence slowly grew and she began talking to her Granddad about the school bullies and standing up for herself when they called her names and pushed her about. This complex story took centre stage in Tom's play therapy for six sessions, and then it simply disappeared. At this time, his mother reported that he no longer displayed extremely high levels of anxiety when going to school and he had independently invited a new friend from school to his house for a play date.

3 Develop feelings of mastery and competence

Puppets were first promoted in therapeutic work with children by Woltmann (1940). He proposed that puppets were useful in therapy, not only because they facilitate self-expression but also because they provide children with opportunities for spontaneity and are easily manipulated. A child can control a puppet, assign its personality, its movements, and expressions. In so doing, puppet play can elicit feelings of mastery and competence, and develop self-confidence and self-efficacy (Tassoni and Hucker, 2005). Puppets can help children manage feelings of insecurity, self-doubt, and low self-esteem. Often, a child holding a puppet manages to do something the child cannot do alone.

Frank, a seven-year-old boy, in his third formal year of school, presented with expressive language difficulties, including a stutter when talking and reading. He displayed poor self-esteem and disliked reading aloud. He received one-to-one resource teaching a number of times each week. His teacher introduced a 'reading puppet' named 'Tommy' who was learning to read aloud. To her amazement, Frank placed the puppet on his hand and read aloud without his stutter. This was the first time in three years that the teacher had heard him speak without the stutter. After a couple of days reading clearly during his one-to-one teaching time, Frank asked could he bring Tommy to meet his class and read for them. Frank proceeded to read aloud, without stuttering, to his entire class.

4 Develop verbal and non-verbal communication

Puppets foster and develop verbal and non-verbal communication (Woodard and Milch, 2012). When an adult manipulates a puppet and brings it to life, the puppet can communicate with the child through gestures, touch, body language, facial expression, eye-contact and words, thus modelling both verbal and non-verbal communication strategies. Similarly, children engage with puppets both verbally and non-verbally. Children laugh when a puppet tells a joke, tries to put his shoe on his hand, or a glove on his foot. They track his movements as he alters his position in the room, reach out to touch him when he moves close to them, and attempt to catch a balloon he throws at them. Children who have difficulty making eye-contact with other people, are often able to make eye-contact with puppets.

I worked with a 4-year-old boy, David, with severe autism, in the classroom environment. When he began school David displayed extremely poor eye-contact, a severe lack of social awareness and responsiveness to others and no desire to interact with his peers. I regularly utilise puppets in my teaching and I immediately noticed that David would look directly at the large puppets that I presented, and even track their movements around the classroom. He displayed an interest in the puppets' actions and communicated joy and engagement through facial expression, eye contact and gestures. In time, David began to transfer these skills to peer relationships.

Clinical applications: practitioner use of puppets

1 Building a puppet profile and other techniques

There are many ways in which the therapist or teacher can use puppets in groupwork, therapy, and educational settings. They may use regular puppets from the playroom to engage a child, develop a fun and healthy connection with the child, model behaviours, role play situations and respond to the child. For example, she (NB I will use 'she' for the adult, and 'he' for the child except when giving specific examples where the adult is male or the child is female) may use a simple technique such as the 'hidden puppet technique' (Bow, 1993) to interact with the child/group of children and support the development of a positive relationship. In this technique the practitioner hides a puppet in a sack, or uses a puppet that can hide in itself, such as a turtle, and encourages the child to help coax the shy puppet out. On other occasions, the therapist or teacher will use a carefully selected puppet and create a personalized profile to engage and address specific issues relevant to a particular child or group of children.

When used by the therapist, the benefits associated with puppets expand further. Narcavagee (1997) presents the idea of using a puppet as a 'symbolic client' in order to engage withdrawn, fearful, and self-conscious children in the beginning stages of therapy. In this technique, the therapist facilitates the projection of the client's feelings onto a puppet and then continues to engage the child in helping to care for the puppet. A therapist may have identified that a client is feeling anxious and scared and thus present a puppet who is feeling scared to the child. The therapist comments on the puppet's emotion and reassures the puppet of its safety. The therapist then moves on to encourage the child to help mind and comfort the frightened puppet. In this approach, the therapist shifts the attention from the child, thus providing dramatic distance and increasing the child's comfort level. Hall *et al.* (2002) believe that using a puppet in this way achieves three essential goals of play therapy: first, the therapist has successfully responded to the child's emotions in a non-threatening fashion; second, the therapist has engaged the child in his therapy; and, third, the collaborative positive therapeutic relationship with the child has begun. In my work with puppets, I have created many puppet profiles both in the classroom and in the therapy room. I believe that the creation of a puppet profile that correlates with the situation, experiences and behaviours of a child is extremely powerful with a wide range of children, not only those who are withdrawn or anxious. A therapist, play specialist or teacher can select and tailor the life, living arrangements, personality, behaviour pattern and temperament of a puppet to suit the needs of a particular child or group. A puppet can be experiencing parental separation, awaiting the arrival of a new sibling, experiencing difficulty with spitting, hitting, kicking, swearing, or can be extremely shy and barely able to talk above a whisper. This type of work requires extensive preparation before introducing the puppet to the client. Even the selection of the appropriate puppet must be carefully considered – male or female, young or old, a mystical character or an animal? For me, the key is selecting a puppet that I feel will appeal to the particular child. Having selected the perfect puppet, the therapist continues to tailor its profile – age, hobbies, personality, family background, personality, temperament etc. – to suit the individual child/group of children before introducing the character into sessions. When using puppets in this way I refer to them as 'friends'. I believe this helps the puppet come to life and illustrates my engagement in the make-believe world of puppetry. Having spent time selecting the appropriate puppet, developing their profile and personality, and ensuring she is comfortable manipulating and using the puppet, the therapist then presents the 'new friend' to the child or group. It is critical not to rush in and use a new puppet before knowing its assigned personality and becoming comfortable manipulating it and speaking to and as it. It is imperative to stay in role. The more comfortable you are in presenting, engaging with the puppet and treating it as if it were real, the more the child will engage with it too. When you are confident that you have done all the relevant preparatory work, it is time to introduce your 'friend' to the child. Your ability to be playful and build up a good story is crucial here. Information and photographs of the 'new friend' can be shared before the puppet even arrives. Letters, postcards, or emails can be sent from the puppet sharing information and expressing a desire to meet. On arrival at the session, the puppet introduces themselves, either by talking directly to the child or whispering in your ear for you to retell, sometimes showing photographs depicting his/her life or sharing a favourite story or toy. The puppet continues to share his/her life experiences; generally this will correlate with the child's situation. In time the child or group of children can be enlisted to give advice to the puppet and help the puppet overcome their particular difficulties. The puppet is not merely used in one introductory session; he/she often becomes an ongoing agent in the child's therapy process. He can attend as many sessions as necessary, until it is apparent that the child no longer needs him. When used in this way, I find that the puppet invariably becomes a friend of the child or the group, someone whom they care for and want to help – no encouragement is needed! On occasion, the puppet will present ideas and new suggestions to the child; for example, he might say how a good friend of his told him to get his parent to put a night light on at bedtime to help stop his bad dreams or that he got a chewy toy to chew on when he feels like eating things that are not safe to eat. Of course, these suggestions will be ideas that I feel may be beneficial to the child. Often when the puppet introduces a new idea or demonstrates a skill, the child is more receptive to it than if I introduce it myself. The puppet and adult can also engage in conversations with each other, within earshot of the child, that are designed to be helpful to the child. The puppet can talk to the practitioner about something that is of concern to the child; for example, talking about a mistaken belief they once held, strong emotions they try to hide or a worry they had. Either the adult or the puppet can present possible solutions within the course of these conversations.

I have witnessed deep bonds emerge between puppets and children. It is necessary to be aware of this and prepare the child for the final goodbye. Remember, the child views the puppet as a real person so it is important for the child to feel that the puppet will miss him/her, too, and for the puppet to be part of the preparations for the final parting. Some strategies that have worked well for me are the creation of memory books, for both the child and the puppet, depicting things they shared and did together, the compilation of a photo album of the child and the puppet, a framed picture of the child and the puppet together for each to keep and a thoughtful card written by the puppet to the child.

2 Psychoeducation

The practice of developing tailored puppet profiles is particularly relevant in the psycheducational component of any intervention, whether this be therapeutic or educational. Psychoeducation is an important component of many psychotherapeutic and educational interventions; it is intended to help a child and/or his parents become more aware of, and better understand, a situation, trauma, condition or behaviour that causes psychological distress. The main goal is to alleviate fears and anxieties and bring about appropriate behavioural change (DeLucia-Waak, 2006). A child may feel anxious, scared or distressed about a current life situation such as parental separation, past trauma (such as sexual abuse), an upcoming event (for example, a hospital appointment) or behaviours he engages in (for example, eating non-edible items). A specifically designed puppet character can have experienced similar traumas or life experiences to the client and can also share the same anxieties, behaviours and coping strategies as the child. They can reach the same crisis points when coping is overwhelmed. This externalisation is extremely beneficial in increasing both child and parental understanding and in normalizing emotions and behaviours (Graham and Reynolds, 2013). When a child better understands the situation, event or behaviour, he is empowered to feel more in control of the situation, thus reducing the stress, fear and anxiety associated with it. In addition, psychoeducation can be used to address cognitive distortions, 'maladaptive patterns of thinking about self, others, and situations, including distortions or inaccurate thoughts (e.g. self-blame for traumatic events) and unhelpful thoughts (e.g. dwelling on the worst possibilities)' (Cohen et al. 2006, p. 23). A therapist-led puppet can be used to challenge cognitive distortions and present new ways of thinking and understanding. Depending on the presenting issue, psychoeducation can be group-based, family-based or individually implemented, by play therapists and/or teachers. Group psychoeducation dealing with issues such as bullying, anger management, parental separation and body image can be used effectively in school settings and creative groupwork programmes both as a preventive measure and as an intervention. Individual and family-based psychoeducation will be most suitable to some clinical issues such as sexual abuse and domestic violence. The psychoeducation component of any intervention is generally focused and goal orientated and includes specific activities designed to target the needs of the child or group (DeLucia-Waak, 2006). In any intervention with children, directive or non-directive, it is imperative that the therapist utilises the child's natural mode of communication – play. The use of puppets, in the psycheducational component of a child's therapy, is a developmentally appropriate, non-threatening and engaging approach. Puppets are extremely effective in raising and exploring sensitive issues with children and their families, teaching new skills and addressing cognitive distortions. Puppets can be used effectively by therapists to act out situations that children fear and help a child understand confusing events. Therapist led puppets can also model and encourage positive interactions and communication, explore new solutions to problems and model conflict resolution. Such interventions allow the child and the therapist to process and alter unhelpful thoughts previously expressed by the child and negative and disruptive behaviours and feelings. In the school setting, I introduce puppets from a range of socio-economic backgrounds, family types and home settings. This ensures all children can relate to the life experiences of at least one puppet. In particular, I have found the use of a puppet from a one-parent home extremely effective in the classroom environment. On numerous occasions I have experienced children from one-parent families, or those currently experiencing parental separation bottling up their feelings and being hesitant to speak about their family.

A number of years ago I was teaching a six-year-old boy, Clive, with Downs Syndrome. Clive's parents were separating at the time. His father had moved out of the family home and Clive and his sister were visiting him in his new home at weekends. Clive had not spoken to me, or anyone else in school, about the changes occurring at home and he still spoke as if his father were living with him. For instance, if recounting an event from the evening before, he would include the father in the story. I decided to introduce 'Sally', a young girl puppet whose father had recently moved out of the family home. Sally had come to me for help as she was feeling sad and confused. As soon as Sally told her story to the children in the class Clive uttered two words, 'same me'. This simple use of Sally had helped to normalize parental separation for Clive. Through Sally, I was able to respond effectively to Clive's verbalisation. In addition, I was able to advise Sally to tell her parents how she was feeling and on strategies to help cheer her up when she was feeling sad. Of course, these strategies were also aimed at Clive, but the use of Sally ensured dramatic distance.

Puppets can be used in similar ways in both group work and individual therapy sessions.

I used a large male puppet in play therapy sessions with Scott. Scott, a six-year-old boy, was referred to play therapy as he had been initiating and engaging in sexually inappropriate behaviour with a younger girl. His parents had reprimanded him seriously and punished him by grounding him. In addition, he was no longer allowed to play with any of his female friends. Scott presented as a caring, energetic, young boy with poor self-esteem and behavioural difficulties. Through his play and conversations with me it became evident that he thought he was a really naughty boy for playing the 'touching game'. It also emerged that he had been exposed to inappropriate, sexually explicit videos. I decided to introduce Scott to 'Alfie', a six-year-old male puppet who had seen kissing and touching on television and didn't really understand what was going on. He was really confused so he tried to figure it out by trying the same behaviour with his sister. His mummy had walked in while he was touching his sister and she was really upset. I then spoke to Alfie and explained that he had tried to do that to his sister because he was confused, he didn't know what he was doing or that it was wrong. He saw something he didn't understand and then he tried to figure it out by doing it to his sister. I explained that touching other children's private body parts and kissing them is not okay, because it is not safe for either child. At the same time, I reiterated that it did not make Alfie a naughty boy, but that it was really important that he didn't do it anymore. Alfie and Scott struck up a friendship and much of my work focused on ensuring the 'touching games' did not happen again, and devising strategies, with them both, that they could use to prevent engaging in the sexualized play again. I believe this technique helped normalize Scott's life experiences, and address his cognitive distortions in a child appropriate manner. I was extremely proud in a later session with Scott and his parents when Scott explained to his parents that his playing the touching games did not make him a naughty boy, just a confused one!

3 Target affective and behavioural dysregulation

The use of a personally designed puppet character is particularly effective in targeting affective and behavioural dysregulation. Affective dysregulation, characterised as 'frequent mood changes and/or difficulty tolerating negative affective states' (Cohen *et al.* 2006, p. 6), refers to a failure to regulate one's emotions effectively (Macklem, 2008). Emotional dysregulation is connected with many of the psychological disorders identified in children and adolescents (Macklem, 2008) and is undoubtedly evident in many of the clients referred for play therapy. It results in poorly modulated emotional responses that often manifest into emotional and behavioural outbursts, displays of aggression towards others, self-harm and a decreased ability to regulate pain (Macklem, 2008). It can lead to behavioural problems such as behavioural dysregulation, relating to both internalizing and externalizing behaviours, and severely impair a child's interpersonal relationships and school performance. A specifically tailored puppet can be used to increase a child's knowledge about emotions and develop awareness of their own feelings and those of others. In addition, such a puppet can be used to teach specific skills such as shifting attention, problem solving, distraction, grounding and self-soothing and regulating techniques, all of which have been identified as central components in the treatment of affective and behavioural dysregulation (Macklem, 2008).

> *Jane, a five-year-old girl presenting with severe attachment disorder, exhibited extremely disruptive behaviours in the classroom environment. She regularly spat, shouted out, cursed, kicked and hit other children and her teacher and engaged in self-harming behaviours. A large female puppet, Mandy, was used extremely effectively in targeting Jane's emotional and behavioural difficulties. I introduced Mandy to the whole class, explained her background and that she needed help with her feelings and her behaviours. She had very mixed-up feelings and because of these she had difficulty with hitting, kicking, spitting etc. Of course the girl chosen (by me) to sit next to Mandy and help her out was Jane! Mandy became a distraction and a soothing tool, and also introduced a range of ideas aimed at promoting self-regulation and thus improving Jane's disruptive behaviours. Mandy introduced a sand box and sensory toys to play with when their hands felt like hurting others or themselves, a chewy toy to chew when they felt like eating crayon and deep breathing and creative visualisations when they felt like they were going to explode! As teacher, I directed my advice on managing feelings and behaviours to both Jane and Mandy, again helping to normalize behaviours and sustain dramatic distance.*

Preventative programs developed specifically to target affective and behavioural dysregulation have proven to be successful when they incorporate problem solving strategies, techniques for coping with anger and when they explore the consequences of behaviour (Macklem, 2008). Therapist-led puppet interventions can be used in individual and group sessions to explore and address all of these issues, in a playful, developmentally appropriate, way.

4 Support storytelling

Storytelling is a powerful therapeutic and educational tool. For the listener, effective storytelling creates a sense of excitement, wonder, mystery and awe. Storytelling fosters a relationship, closeness and sharing between teller and listener (Collins and Cooper, 1997). In addition, storytelling has the ability to be both informative and non-threatening. Stories create dramatic distance and thus can present a wide range of psychological messages, concepts and ideas for children. As a result, the technique of telling therapeutic stories, for example those by Sunderland (2000) and Davis (1985), can be very successful in educating, treating and healing a range of psychological difficulties. The inclusion of puppets as a storytelling tool helps the storyteller introduce stories in a playful, warm manner. When a puppet known to a child introduces his favourite story it immediately engages the child's interest and makes the story more meaningful and relevant. The use of a puppet as a character within a story helps bring the tale to life and to maintain the child's interest and attention. The child travels on the same journey as the character they identify with, experiencing the same highs and lows, frustrations and solutions. In addition, they are no longer alone – the character shares their situation (Sunderland, 2000) and successful resolutions in the story bring hope to the child. The more engaging the story, the more likely the child is to adopt the concepts, ideas and messages within it. The use of a puppet as a character within a story also allows for the development of its storyline. The child can ask the puppet questions about what happened next, and give the puppet advice and help. In addition, the puppet can introduce more focused activities relating to the theme.

5 Ensure fun and playfulness take centre stage in creative groupwork

Creative groupwork with children can be extremely effective as both a treatment and a preventative measure. The puppet techniques outlined above relating to 'symbolic clients', puppet profiles, psychoeducation, targeting affective and behavioural regulation, and storytelling can effectively be incorporated into any groupwork intervention. One of the main difficulties that can arise for group facilitators is successfully balancing the recognition of the individual and the provision of freedom to express oneself and present emotionally relevant material with managing group behaviours to ensure the group runs smoothly and offers safety and containment for all. Creative groupwork requires a clear structure and rules so that fun and playfulness can be facilitated within a safe space. Puppets are effective tools in setting up group routines, rules, and boundaries and promoting positive behaviours and interactions (Bentley, 2005). In groupwork situations, puppets can be used to help draw up contracts stating group rules. For example, a specific puppet can invite the children to suggest the rules they think are important for the group. This puppet can reframe the suggested rules in a positive light, such as changing 'no hitting' to 'We use gentle touch in the group'. This specific puppet can be reintroduced at the start of each session to remind the children of the group rules/contract and can be brought out at any stage during sessions if the leader feels any of the rules need to be reinforced. A puppet can also be used to address social skill deficits in group situations. A puppet with disruptive behaviours, such as aggressive outbursts, inability to share materials, poor attention and listening skills, can join a group and the group can be in charge of teaching the puppet new behaviours. Children generally relish showing a disruptive puppet how to take turns, share materials and listen to others – behaviours a group intervention might aim to foster. Using a puppet in this way shifts the attention away from the disruptive behaviour of the children and provides opportunities for the group leader to acknowledge and praise the child for engaging in positive behaviours, thus reinforcing these behaviours rather than the negative ones. In addition, the simple act of entrusting the children to help the puppet and take on the teacher role can increase self-confidence and feelings of self-worth. Throughout the sessions the puppet can share stories, activities and games with the children. He can introduce new concepts and ideas, in a fun and friendly way, thus ensuring the educational component of groupwork is relevant, engaging and playful.

Choosing puppets for the playroom

In order to ensure children have the opportunity to express a range of emotions and experiences, it is essential to include a wide variety of puppets in the playroom (DeLucia-Waak, 2006). This includes people puppets of varying ages, genders, and cultures; animal puppets ranging from quiet, timid animals such as rabbits and tortoises to more aggressive animals such as lions and tigers; mystical creatures such as dragons and mermaids; and specific character puppets such as doctors and fire-fighters. It is also important to consider the size of puppets; some children will be drawn to large puppets, while others will prefer smaller glove or sleeve puppets and finger puppets. The puppets can be displayed on a puppet stand, hung on the back of a door, laid out on shelves or simply kept in a large basket or box. In addition, simple puppet making materials should be provided in the playroom. Children can easily make sock puppets, paper plate puppets, wooden spoon puppets and finger puppets with a simple selection of junk art materials. Specific puppets for therapist use, as characters with personalized profiles, are separate from regular playroom puppets as they will only be introduced with specific clients. However, some of the standard puppets can also have more general characteristics associated with them (for example, the wise owl, the wizard with magic powers, the sly fox, the timid mouse) and can be available for the child to use in their spontaneous play. Generally speaking, I use large boy and girl puppets or large animal puppets when using a puppet as a symbolic client. Children generally relate extremely well to the boy and girl puppets, build up a strong relationship with them and are very eager to help them out. Animal or mystical puppets can create more dramatic distance, so if you are worried that a child will shut down and think you are just mimicking them then it may be best to use a large animal puppet or a mystical character instead of a boy/girl puppet. When creating profiles for animal or mystical puppets, I also create a home for them to live in and appear from – a decorated shoebox, a wicker basket, a cloth bag, a kennel etc. I believe the creation of the home adds to the magic and sense of occasion when I first introduce the puppet and makes the characters more believable. I do not create homes for my large people puppets, as I believe they should live in houses, apartments or mobile homes, not boxes – they are people after all! Instead, I have the puppet tell about his home and share photographs of it.

Conclusion

In this chapter, I have shared with you a range of my experiences of using puppets in both therapeutic and educational settings. I have outlined many of the reasons why puppets are so effective when working with children, and presented a multitude of benefits associated with puppet use. In addition, clinical techniques and applications, addressing both the child's use and the therapist's use of puppets, have been outlined, thus highlighting the crucial role puppets serve in play therapy. Issues surrounding choosing puppets, equipping your playroom and using puppets appropriately have also been explored, and the importance of feeling comfortable using puppets highlighted. So now that the reading is done, it is time to pop a puppet on and get practising. Enjoy!

Key points

1. Puppets are naturally engaging and can serve a crucial role in therapeutic and educational settings.
2. Puppets can be used effectively by both the therapist and the child.
3. Child's use of puppets fosters and promotes the expression of thoughts and feelings, development of understanding and insights, release of fears, worries and aggression, development of

feelings of mastery and competence, and verbal and non-verbal communication.
4. A therapist may use regular puppets from the playroom to engage a child, develop a fun and healthy connection with the child, model behaviours, role play situations and respond to the child's puppets.
5. Therapists can also use puppets in a more focused way when addressing psychoeducation, targeting affective and behavioural regulation, creating and telling therapeutic stories and managing groups.
6. In order to ensure children have the opportunity to express a range of emotions and experiences, it is essential to include a wide variety of puppets in the playroom.

References

Astell-Burt, C. (2002). *I Am the Story: The art of puppetry in education and therapy*. UK: The Guernsey Press Co. Ltd.
Bentley, L. (2005). *Puppets at Large: Puppets as partners in learning and teaching in the Early Years*. UK: Positive Press Ltd.
Bow, J. N. (1993). Overcoming resistance. In C. E. Schaefer (ed.), *The Therapeutic Powers of Play* (pp. 17–40). Northvale, NJ: Jason Aronson.
Cohen, J. A., Mannarino, A. P. and Deblinger, E. (2006). *Treating Trauma and Traumatic Grief in Children and Adolescents*. New York, NY: Guilford Press.
Collins, R. and Cooper, P. J. (1997). *The Power of Story: Teaching through storytelling*. Long Grove, IL: Waveland Press, Inc.
Davis, N. (1985). *Therapeutic Stories to Heal Abused Children*. Oxon Hill, MD: Psychological Associates of Oxon Hill.
DeLucia-Waack, J. L. (2006). *Leading Psychoeducational Groups for Children and Adolescents*. USA: Sage Publications.
Engler, L. and Fijan, C. (1973). *Making Puppets Come Alive: How to learn and teach hand puppetry*. New York: Dover Publications Inc.
Featherstone, S. and MacDonald, S. (2005). *The Little Book of Puppets in Stories: Little books with big ideas*. UK: Featherstone Education Ltd.
Graham, P. and Reynolds, S. (2013). *Cognitive Behaviour Therapy for Children and Families*. Cambridge: Cambridge University Press.
Hall, T. M., Kaduson, H. G. and Schaefer, C. E. (2002). Fifteen effective play therapy techniques. *Professional Psychology: Research and practice*, 33 (6), 515–522.
Jennings, S. (2008). *Creative Puppetry with Children and Adults*. UK: Speechmark.
Kaduson, H. and Schaefer, C. (eds) (1997). *101 Favorite Play Therapy Techniques*. Northvale, NJ: Jason Aronson.

Kaduson, H. G. and Schaefer, C. (eds) (2001). *101 More Favorite Play Therapy Techniques*. Northvale, NJ: Jason Aronson.

Law, M. B. (2004). Set the stage. *ASCA School Counsellor*, 41, 14–19.

Macklem, G. L. (2008). *Practitioner's Guide to Emotion Regulation in School-Aged Children*. New York, NY: Springer.

Narcavagee, C. J. (1997). Using a puppet to create a symbolic client. In H. Kaduson and C. Schaefer (eds) (1997), *101 Favorite Play Therapy Techniques* (pp. 199–203). Northvale, NJ: Jason Aronson.

Sunderland, M. (2000). *Using Storytelling as a Therapeutic Tool with Children*. London: Speechmark.

Tassoni, P. and Hucker, K. (2005). *Planning Play and the Early Years*. UK: Pearson Education Ltd.

Thorp, G. (2005). *The Power of Puppets*. UK: Positive Press Ltd.

VanSchuvver, J. M. (1993). *Storytelling Made Easy with Puppets*. Phoenix, AZ: Orxy Press.

Woltmann, A. G. (1940). The use of puppets in understanding children. *Mental Hygiene*, 24, 445–458.

Woodard, C. and Milch, C. (2012). *Make-Believe Play and Story-Based Drama in Early Childhood: Let's pretend!* London: Jessica Kingsley Publishers.

7 Working therapeutically with groups in the outdoors
A natural space for healing

Maggie Fearn

Introduction

> The body is the medium through which we experience ourselves and the environment.
>
> (Olsen, 2002, p. xxi)

This chapter proposes that we do well to consider including the natural environment as a significant presence in the therapeutic relationship and as a fundamental pre-requisite for integrated sensory-motor development. As well as introducing some somatic theory, it includes games and activities that link the sensory and perceptive experience of the moving body with the elements and life forms contained in the surrounding environment. The exploratory mode is kinaesthetic and is primarily experiential. As children become familiar with the outdoor space, with the practitioner's presence and the materials and play opportunities that we develop together, they gradually begin to find their ground and experience relationship with the natural world. Focussing attention on dynamic interaction with the environing space has powerful therapeutic potential.

Embodying the environment

A child is born into an environment of sensation, learning to orientate herself through attachment to significant sensory experiences, which include the presence of her primary caregiver (Bowlby, 1969), the character and atmosphere of her home environment and transitional objects, sounds and textures. She is developing a relationship with her environment that is full of signifiers (Winnicott, 2005; Cyrulnik, 1993). For her, their meanings are intrinsically about survival and growth, and she seeks acknowledgement and response in a process of adaptation and integration as her experience and understanding of the world develops. Cozolino (2002) describes healthy attachment as a process of the caregiver's attunement and resonance with the infant's internal states, and the ability of the caregiver to translate the child's experience into actions and words appropriate to the child's stage of development. This gives the child the ability to connect internal states with expressive movement, action, sound and, eventually, language. In relationship, she develops the ability to receive sensory information, regulate and manage incoming sensations and respond within a comfortable range of arousal. Formed like the webbing of a root system, her whole nervous system can adjust to simultaneous stimuli without going into survival mode.

With good enough attachment, children will interact with their environment and all it contains through the medium of exploration and play (Landreth, 2002). At the heart of play is the individual child's experience and what that feels like. 'When the sensory developmental supports in the child's environment are missing, the world no longer has an outline' (Cyrulnik, 2005: 13). Research suggests that poor attachment with primary caregivers causes emotional distress, with predictions of long-term effects on a child's ability to develop healthy relationships. A child who is hurt or neglected by her caregivers has often shut down her sensory explorations and lives in fear, resulting in poor body awareness (Cattanach, 1997). Gerhardt (2004) describes the sensitive stress response, a state in which the child cannot self-regulate because of the constant hyper arousal that results from unmet needs, or the hypo vigilant state of withdrawal and depression that results from giving up. However, Jennings (2011) suggests that therapeutic play can help these children because, over the lifespan, neural plasticity allows for, and benefits from, the healing effects of a sensitive therapeutic relationship that endures over time.

Lester and Russell summarize research findings about neural plasticity and its development through flexible play behaviour, saying 'While guided and framed by genetic information, a great deal of neural patterning occurs through the child's interaction with her or his environment (often referred to as experience dependent plasticity)' (2008, pp. 3 and 10). When knowledge is needed, we draw on previous experiences, which are laid down in our neural systems in categories. These experiences are reactivated to simulate how the body previously reacted to similar sensory stimuli. Grounded cognition theory explores the significance of simulation based on embodied experience (Barsalou, 2008). It is suggested that our neurological systems evolve through situated action, which emphasizes the inter-relationship between an action and its context: our perception, emotional state, physical body, the environment, and other actors, including social interaction. The more present and aware we are for the original experience, the more complete the simulation will be.

A characteristic of play is the intensity of, and absorption in, the present moment. Children are preoccupied when they play and are not normally 'compliant or acquiescent' to influences outside the frame of play (Winnicott, 2005, p. 68). Playful experiences are deeply impressive: the playing child is engaged in physiological interaction through sensory connection with her environment and all it contains. From an early age, a child seeks dialogue with her environment. She meets the world in open sensory attention, much as E. O. Wilson (1984) describes the hunter-naturalist's mode of being: in full attention, avoiding inattention, taking in a wide field of detail. She is not focussed on consistency but is alert for the unexpected, responding to the environment's myriad expressions of life. She is thinking with the body, attuned to sensory information and inviting reciprocity with an animated landscape. This engenders a sense of agency and identity, inner and outer worlds meeting in co-responsive attention.

Natural environments provide experiences of connection with other life forms, like insect, mammal, tree, wind, rock, soil, water, flower, light, the sun's heat, the coolness of rain and shade, providing 'experiences of identity with elements out of which human life in fact comes' (Chawla, 2009, p. 209). They provide optimum play spaces, full of richness and abundance to feed and stimulate the senses, encouraging absorption and extended play, and providing interactive experiences in nature that expand a child's conceptual framework (Kellert, 2002).

As they play, children construct narratives rooted in their lived experience, flowing back and forth between fantasy and reality in a way most adults have lost (Cattanach, 2001).

> It was noticeable that, when the children played alone, particularly when absorbed in movement, as for example when hanging upside down from a branch, they would often be talking to themselves in a stream of narrative. During play, action and language merged in a creative flow. Vygotsky (1978) observed that in young children action always precedes language.... Embodied experience appears to structure thought rather than thought structuring experience as in adolescence and adulthood. For a young child, to construct a thought is to associate embodied experience with sensory response to the immediate context/environment. For example:
> Child: *'I like brushing the trees (with a paintbrush and water) because it helps them grow, and itch.'* Researcher: *'How does it help*

them grow?' Child: *'When it itches a lot and looks like it's having a bath.'*

This child associates his actions in the present moment with embodied memory of the relief of water on itchy skin. Vygotsky proposes that 'memory in early childhood is one of the central psychological functions upon which all other functions are built' (1978, p. 50).

(Fearn and North, 2010)

Children embody their environment, creating patterns of response through a process of movement of attention, absorbing or defending against sensory information and forming perception (Bainbridge Cohen, 2008). The imprint of trauma can inhibit or prevent the completion of this loop. Encouraging a child to become absorbed in sensory play in nature can override defensive patterns and restore a whole and integrated sensory pathway, enabling her to draw full benefit from a dynamic relationship with the natural environment, and to respond through symbolic play with natural and found materials.

The outdoors as therapeutic play space

Sensory immersion and assimilation of the surrounding world under effective conditions of well being and security in which the child can peacefully and playfully be at one with its body and the world.

(Kahn and Kellert, 2002, p. 213)

The natural world exists in community: rocks, streams, soil, plants, trees and creatures living off and with each other in synchronised, reciprocal arrangements that have evolved over many generations of adaptation and cooperation, in light, shade and darkness. Ancient woodlands, that once covered most of the UK, provide us with experience of a complex ecosystem and often have evidence of current and historical management that brings humans into the natural community in a way that cooperates with, rather than dominates, the environment. These are elemental places where children can play naturally.

Not everyone can access woodland, but it is presented here as the optimum against which to assess other spaces. Perhaps a garden or parkland is within reach. Nothing too tidy! Consider the natural community: are there trees, shrubs, perennial plants, areas of wildness, long grass and wild flowers, rough bits of ground, deadwood on the ground, humps and tussocks, places to hide, to rest, to run and climb? It needs to be private, with no through traffic of the human variety. Consider the area you will be using and be clear about its boundaries.

A word about safety

There is a balance to be struck between children's vital need for risk and challenge and adult concerns for their safety. It helps to weigh up the benefit of an activity against the perceived risk. Therapeutic practitioners need to use their knowledge of the environment, the children and the particular circumstances in an ongoing process of assessment that places each child's interests and motivations at the heart of decision-making. In most cases, children can be trusted to learn to assess and take manageable risks for themselves and it is vital for the development of self-other awareness that they do so.

Children will explore and experiment as they play and, as a rule of thumb, the outdoors environment needs to be assessed for hazards that may cause serious injury; such as, for example, dangerous litter, holes in the ground where they may run, poisonous plants they may pick and eat, dead branches they may hang from or climb on and spiky eye level branches. Children need to learn about these things. Some, such as litter or dead and spiky branches where children play, can be removed or made safe; others, like holes and plants, can be marked and the children told about them.

But let us also look at the benefits: for example, deadwood is home to myriad creatures that are creating the soil that keeps us alive. Children need to know this, it is their right to know it, and so deadwood has a place in their play environment. Holes in the ground are evidence that this special place is someone else's home. Plants that are poisonous to humans support other life forms and have a right to life themselves. Children need to know this, too, and learn the identification skills that can preserve their own life and the life of plant and creature, thus participating in the natural community.

Resources

Children will discover, and interact with, what is there. In therapeutic outdoor play they are given permission to move in close relationship between earth and sky: to be belly flat on the ground, to roll, creep and crawl, to climb and swing. They need to be dressed appropriately, in strong shoes, lightweight waterproof over-trousers and old clothes.

In order not to deplete the site's natural materials, and to create opportunities for extended play that bridges inner and outer worlds, it will be necessary to build up resources that may include some or all of the following, packed so that everything has its place, clearly marked:

- sticks of differing lengths and diameters – for example willow whips, hazel rods, ash staffs and elder wands
- stones of different sizes, colours and weights
- balls of wool and string
- small world people
- woodland creature puppets
- clay
- water
- tracking and species ID books
- bug boxes
- nets, ropes, small tarpaulins, hammocks and swings
- simple rhythm instruments, chimes
- compass
- small baskets
- pots, spoons, tongs, tweezers and brushes
- trowels

The sessions

Therapeutic outdoor play sessions are intended to nurture small groups of children aged from four to eleven years. They may know each other a little; for example, they may go to the same school or nursery. They may have been referred as individuals who would benefit from group experiences. Sometimes children flourish in mixed age groups, sometimes they need peer group experiences. Family sessions can give parents and care givers valuable insights into the importance of playing with their children outdoors and the skills to support their children's play.

Ideally, the therapeutic play practitioner provides a calm, embodied presence. There are tensions between the non-directive facilitation of children's play experiences and the desire to introduce ideas that may support a child's process. It is a fine balance to find ways of introducing any games and activities in a way that responds to the child's play interests, rather than directs them. There is vital skill in being able to both hold the group with your full attention and relax sufficiently into the background. It helps to check in with your own responses. If you find yourself playing, then acknowledge that you need to play, but elsewhere, not in the session.

If you find yourself directing, take a step back and allow the direction of the group. Pay attention to your own felt senses as you work, and learn to modulate your responses. Don't rush anyone, ever – we need to give children the space and time to discover their innate patterns and pacing. This is the most precious gift.

The activities are offered as resources to be used sensitively to enrich and enliven an outdoors play space. It may be that we play a game together, and something in the game inspires the children's next move. Forget the game. Follow the children! Stay with them, respond and they will let you know what they need you to do.

Sessions typically begin with one hour on site and, over time, when the children are ready, can extend to two hours. It is recommended that the practitioner initiates the session with an activity and, after that, themes evolve in response to the children's developing play. Five to ten minutes before the end of the session, bring the group together for sharing, feedback and planning for the next session. Establishing a routine at the start and end of each session provides a secure framework signalling the parameters of the session and offering a sense of containment that supports the evolution of the group.

Location, orientation and creating a hearth

The hearthstone is a powerful symbol of 'home'. Creating a hearth as a place to return to, to share by, to travel out from, gives the children a centre of belonging. It will manifest the intentions for the group: a place of beauty, calm, and safety. It can be decorated each session, reflecting the energetic and elemental themes that are emerging from the group.

> Our first question is not: Who am I? It is: Where am I?
>
> (Straus, 1966)

We explore that which orientates and supports us. We call this Sensory Mapping and we begin with boundaries. In somatic understanding, our felt sense boundary is our skin and then, moving outwards, into our kinaesthetic field of awareness. A boundary is always a meeting place where an exchange can occur through touch between self and other. In nature this exchange occurs without the complexity of human relationship. Ground touches foot, wind touches skin, sound touches hearing, aroma touches olfactory nerve. Children are given time and space to be touched by nature and to allow an exchange, leaving both human and elemental affected by the meeting.

Matching ribbons

You will need:

- A compass
- 4 sets of 10 to12 ribbons in 5–6 different hues of the primaries: blue, yellow, green and red.

Before the session orientate yourself to compass North. Mark the North boundary in an arc with 5–6 well-spaced different shades of blue ribbons, all of which can be seen from a central point (the boundary can change and move outwards after a few sessions, as the group becomes securely grounded and orientated). Then mark East with 5–6 yellow hues; South with 5–6 red hues; West with 5–6 green hues. Try to space them so they meet and a boundary is marked in a circle of graded colours around the site.

Give the children the compass to locate North and discuss with them the four directions and the colour system (e.g. What does North feel like? Is blue the right colour?). Give each child a set of the remaining ribbons, which as a group they take to the boundary and match colour to colour, tying their ribbons to the others. When all the ribbons have been matched to each other, return to the hearth as a group.

As we return, we explore who or what might live within the boundary, and perhaps find evidence of creatures who may be coming and going. We might also talk about swallows and salmon, finding their way back to their breeding grounds, over thousands of miles, guided by the sun and sea and air currents. The children become aware of outer boundaries and limits as spatial concepts related to creature instinct and habit. They are orientating to space and ground.

Beating the bounds (traditional)

You will need:

- a selection of rattles and shakers, enough for each child to have one.

In one group, the children set up a rhythm and rattle and shake around the boundary. On our return to the starting point, we stop and listen to the stunned silence of the natural world and the gradual return of small sounds.

At the hearth we talk about a boundary as a ring of protection. We ask the children to close their eyes and imagine their very own boundary: what is it made of?

For integration, provide art materials for each child to make an image of their boundary.

Create a map of recognisable features showing what is contained within the site and what is on the margins, and at the end of each session encourage the children to add symbols for their experiences on the map. Recognising and mapping boundaries and limits in the shared outer world, and what happens within them, awakens awareness of the possibility of a rich inner world with safe boundaries.

Awareness is learnt, it is selective; it is about focussing attention (Hanna, 1970).

Sound mapping

Children 5+ can play this game on their own, younger children may need a helper. Explain this is a listening game: to hear like a fox or a bat we can cup our hands behind our ears to hear what is in front of us; and to hear what is behind, cup them on the front of the ears facing backwards (Cornell, 1989).

Encourage each child to find their special place within earshot of you, and explain we can hear better if our eyes are closed, but you don't have to – some children are afraid of closing their eyes at first. Explain that the game says to stay in one place and listen very carefully for sounds all around them. Begin with paying attention to faraway sounds for a minute, then bring their attention into the middle ground ... then close by ... then listening for sounds from within their own bodies. Move their attention out again, to the immediate surroundings, then to the middle ground, then to sounds far away. Offer a few minutes for the children to explore sounds unguided. To finish, bring their attention into the group by tinkling a small bell. Call everyone back to the hearth and share experiences with each other.

Children become deeply absorbed in sound mapping. It is unusual to be in a place where machines and other human sounds cannot be heard – how beautiful if you can find that peace! If not, it can be helpful for children to learn to differentiate natural sounds from machines; we often find that children cannot make that distinction. Once that difference is understood, they can begin to differentiate sound from sound in the natural world – the details of different bird songs, the whisper of a breeze through leaves, the gurgle and splosh of water, the hum and buzz of insects. Differentiation heightens awareness of our sensory world, bringing us into the present moment. Learning to identify where a sound is coming from, anchors a child in her body. Here I am! I am a listener!

This activity plays with fields of perception. It gives the children an opportunity to explore closeness and distance, to find their comfort zone and rest there. Vision is the last in the sensory developmental sequence and integrates movement, touch, smell and hearing (Bainbridge Cohen, 2008). We live in a culture that is dominated by visual information. The relationship between head, neck and eye is commonly over strained. Cupping the ears soothes the cranial nerves and paying attention to the hearing sense rebalances and reminds the eyes they can rest.

The Talking Stick

You will need:

- a wand of hazel, comfortable to hold, perhaps imprinted with a honeysuckle spiral, if you are lucky enough to find one
- a small basket of colored threads.

At times when we are sat around the hearth sharing our experiences, we use the Talking Stick.

Whoever is holding the Talking Stick holds the Power to Speak. Those who are not holding the Talking Stick have the Power to Listen. They give their full attention because they know it will be their turn soon. There is an understanding that everyone in the group has something of equal value to offer. As each child finishes speaking they select a coloured thread from the basket and tie it onto the stick, then pass it on to the next speaker.

Holding the Talking Stick can give a child the power of speech. It may not happen at once. A child may hold the stick wordlessly many times. The others use their special Power to Listen and often hear what cannot be spoken and, gradually, over time, the words find their way out into the safety of the shared hearth space.

Magic potions

You will need:

- knowledge of what is growing on the site!
- a selection of different smells
- cups or pots
- water
- a paintbrush for each child and mixing sticks.

NB Safety considerations: mark and show the children anything you don't want them to touch, and explain why.

Each child has a pot with a little water in it and a paintbrush. Suggest the children explore the site by painting smells. By first painting something with water, then sniffing it, each child selects a sample of smells they like. You can also provide for example: aromatic plants, oranges, rose petals.... It is an absorbing activity, the ritual of painting and smelling calms and soothes. Then they can mix a potion in their pot from their favourite smells. Encourage them to find words for each smell as they add it to their pot.

Our sense of smell is not mediated through the spinal cord; an aroma passes directly up the nose and into the brain. 'The olfactory nerves are the only cranial nerves attached directly to the cerebrum' (Martini, 2006, p. 481). Finding words for smells brings attention to the process of perception and embodied memory. Attention integrates past experiences in relation to the present conditions.

The ground beneath our feet

Our feet connect us to the ground. Through the ground we are connected to our life support, the plants and the trees, and they communicate with each other through air via pollinators, and through their roots via an underground mesh of fungi, which enable them to share resources. We are part of a complex and cooperative natural community.

A short visualisation

With eyes closed, we imagine we are all trees, we bring our attention to our feet and feel every inch of our feet in contact with the ground ... gradually, small roots start to grow from the soles of our feet into the earth beneath. The roots are like hair, but they are strong and they know how to find their way down through the particles of soil, in amongst the soil creatures, and millions of other hair roots, down through the clay and stones to the great rock caverns deep beneath us.... Gradually the roots thicken and become strong enough for us to grow upwards towards the sun, raising our arms as branches to capture the sunlight through our leaves. Imagine your leaves, their color and shape. Imagine the flowers of your tree and the seeds that fly away in the wind, whilst you stay firmly, strongly, deeply rooted to the ground. Now imagine a child leaning against the trunk of your tree....

> Let yourself become that child, resting, feeling safe and comfortable leaning against the trunk of your favourite tree. Feel the strong tree against your back. Feel the sunlight as it shines down on you through the branches of your beautiful tree.... Rest, knowing you are safe and that your tree will always be there. Slowly begin to move and stretch your body ... cup your hands over your eyes, then open your eyes, getting used to the light.
>
> For integration, provide art materials for children to make images of their tree.
>
> Proprioception is the movement sense that integrates incoming sensations to tell us where we are. This visualization supports organization in the vertical, seeking equal support from space (reaching up towards the sun) and ground (reaching down deep into the earth). Integral to the activity is the developmental movement pattern of yielding to find support (against our special tree), feeling trust in our environment (the internal world of imagination) and allowing an approach from outside towards the self (from sunlight). The natural world allows this process, it is animated other, yet non-human.

Movement and imagination

Being upright is just one of many possible relationships with the ground yet, like vision, it dominates our culture. Left to explore freely, very young children will experience a variety of different movement patterns that bring them into the vertical as just one of many possibilities. Reminding the body of its potential for a variety of movement releases tensions held deep in the musculature, and liberates the imagination. Here are some suggestions that encourage a range of movement in association with sensory play.

Playing with footsteps 1 – Human feet

You will need:

- water
- bare earth
- clay.

1. Create a mud play area and 'wellysplosh' in it, making footsteps, following in each other's, jumping, squelching. Find ways to make mudprints – large sheets perhaps, or cardboard.
2. Make tablets of clay and imprint bare feet. Compare each other's imprints. Make a footprint gallery.

Playing with footsteps 2 – Animal/bird feet

You will need:

- magnifiers and bug pots
- a tracking ID book.

1. Search the site for evidence of footprints of other creatures.
2. Search for insects in damp dark places. Use magnifying bug pots and handle the creatures as little as possible – our hands are hot for a bug! Notice how many legs they have – can you see their feet? Imagine their tiny footprints and make imprints with twigs on clay tablets. We always return the creatures to where we find them – they have homes and families, too.

Playing with footsteps 3 – Imaginary creatures' feet

You will need:

- clay
- things you find on the ground such as moss, sticks, earth, flowers, leaves etc.
- connecting and tying materials such as gardening string, raffia, ivy strands.

Imagine the footprints of a fairy, a monster, a giant, an elf, a fabulous creature, something from your imagination ... start with the feet and create the owner of those feet!

String stories: crawling, being close to the ground

Children can work alone or in pairs.
You will need:

- about 3 feet of string per child
- clay.

Each child, or pair, finds a place of their own and lays the string along the ground: it may lay across holes, sticks, branches, over and under plants, across a tree trunk, through a puddle.

Imagining being as small as an insect, the children create little creatures from clay and found materials and they take them on a journey along their string, overcoming obstacles, meeting enemies and helpers, making friends and helping others along the way, until they arrive at their destination. After 10–15 minutes, making time, we move from one string story to the next, hearing about the adventures of the tiny heroes and heroines.

Rope and net, blanket and hammock: rolling, down and up, dizzy play, resting, tumbling

Here are a few more suggestions for making spaces to explore different ways of moving in the world:

- Designate an area for lying on your backs, looking up through the trees to the sky above.
- Encourage slow rolling on blankets laid out on open ground.
- Set up a slack rope for balancing on by fixing thick ropes between strong trees – the lower rope about 18 inches off the ground, the higher one above head height for reaching up and holding on to.
- Set up hammocks for individuals to take time out. Actively encourage children to know when they need to rest.
- Provide den-building materials. Children will express their individuality, set their boundaries and create a space that feels truly their own.
- Set up large nets, tied securely between four sturdy trees. Children will use them for group quiet time, and rough and tumble play.

Set up a simple swing. Children seek disequilibrium in their play; it allows them to explore the boundaries of being in and out of control (Olsen 2002).

Conclusion

This chapter has briefly introduced a somatic approach to therapeutic outdoor play and provides support and guidance for therapeutic practitioners who are considering taking children outside. Working therapeutically outdoors with groups of children needs a combination of specialist skills and knowledge. These can be summed up in an attitude of relaxed attention that holds simultaneous awareness of the group's and individual needs, underpinned by trust in the power of play and acknowledgement of the natural environment as a significant presence in the therapeutic process. During the sessions the group evolves through reciprocal relationships – child to environment, child to child, child to adult, adult to environment – in an ongoing process of co-creation.

> The group has been coming to the wood for a few weeks, and each child is beginning to settle in. The treasure hunt was a child's proposal and we focus on children's perceptions of what it might be. We asked: 'What is treasure?' The children say: 'leaves' and 'feathers'. They also find special pieces of wood, bark and moss.
>
> (Fearn and North, 2010)

Out of the initial idea, a range of different activities emerged, such as making maps, and mark making on trees using cold charcoal from the fire; threading leaves on sticks; and digging, burying and hiding things. Each child was absorbed for the whole session, their personal narratives expressed through their play. Although the group never came together in a conventional way to 'do' a treasure hunt, it was clear from their original intention, and their shared understandings at the end of the session, that everything each child did, alone or with others, also had a collective meaning. Therapeutic outdoor play with groups succeeds when it encourages simultaneously the felt senses of individual expression and group belonging.

A grounded child is absorbed in the present moment, held by gravity between earth and sky, moving freely in response to sensory information from her environment. A child who fully senses who she is in relationship to a special person, and where she is in relationship with a special place, has the inner resources that will support her adolescent curiosity to discover who she is in relationship to other places and other people.

Key points

1. Somatic theory explains how playing in a natural environment can support children's development and resilience.
2. Simple ideas can support immersion in the natural world and facilitate sensory awareness.
3. The natural environment is an inherently therapeutic place.

References

Bainbridge Cohen, B. (2008). *Sensing Feeling and Action: The Experiential Anatomy of Body-Mind Centering* (2nd edn). Northampton, MA: Contact Editions.

Barsalou, L. W. (2008). Grounded Cognition. *Annual Review of Psychology*, 59, 617–645.

Bowlby, J. (1969). *Attachment and Loss*. Volume 1. London: Hogarth Press.

Cattanach, A. (1997). *Children's Stories in Play Therapy*. London: Jessica Kingsley Publications.

Chawla, L. (2002). Spots of Time: Manifold Ways of Being in Nature in Childhood. In P. Kahn and S. Kellert, *Children and Nature: Psychological, Sociocultural and Evolutionary Investigations* 8 (pp. 199–225). USA: MIT.

Cornell, J. (1989). *Sharing Nature with Children II*. Nevada, CA: Dawn Publications.

Cozolino, L. (2002). *The Neuroscience of Psychotherapy*. London: Norton. Cited in S. Jennings (2011). *Healthy Attachments and Neurodramatic Play*. London: Jessica Kingsley Publications.

Cyrulnik, B. (1993). *The Dawn of Meaning*. New York: McGraw Hill.

Cyrulnik, B. (2005). *Speaking of Love on the Edge of a Precipice*. London: Allen Lane

Fearn, M. and North, S. (2010). Validating Child-led Free Play in the Context of Forest School: Play Based Pedagogy and Children's Perspectives (unpublished). PDF available from info@movementsense.co.uk

Gerhardt, S. (2004). *Why Love Matters. How affection shapes a baby's brain*. New York: Routledge.

Hanna, T. (1997). *Bodies in Revolt. A Primer in Somatic Thinking*. USA: Holt, Rhinhart and Winston.

Jennings, S. (2011). *Healthy Attachments and Neurodramatic Play*. London: Jessica Kingsley Publications.

Kahn, P. and Kellert, S. (2002). *Children and Nature: Psychological, Sociocultural and Evolutionary Investigations* 5 (pp. 117–152). USA: MIT.

Kellert, S. (2002). Experiencing Nature: Affective, Cognitive and Evaluative Development in Children. In P. Kahn and S. Kellert, *Children and Nature: Psychological, Sociocultural and Evolutionary Investigations* 5 (pp. 117–152). USA: MIT.

Landreth, G. (2002). *Play Therapy. The Art of the Relationship* (2nd edn). New York: Brunner Routledge.

Lester, S. and Russell, W. (2008). *Play for a Change*. London: National Children's Bureau.

Martini, F. (2006). *Fundamentals of Anatomy and Physiology*. USA: Pearson Benjamin Cummings.

Olsen, A. (2002). *Body and Earth: An Experiential Guide*. NH: Middlebury College Press.

Straus, E. (1966). *Phenomenological Psychology*. London: Tavistock Publications.

Vygotsky, L. (1978). *Mind in Society*. Cambridge, MA: Harvard University Press.
Wellhöfer, K. and Fearn, M. (2011). Somatic Skills for Practitioners across Contexts. Paper presented at Wellbeing 2010 Conference Birmingham University. PDF available from info@movementsense.co.uk
Wilson, E. O. (1984). *Biophilia*. Cambridge MA: Harvard University Press.
Winnicott, D. W. (2005). *Playing and Reality*. Oxford: Routledge Classics.

8 Group play therapy for children with multiple disabilities

Eimir McGrath

Introduction

The value of play therapy interventions for children with intellectual disabilities has received little attention in the current literature, yet even the most profoundly disabled child has the capacity for an active emotional life that can be enhanced through experiencing a therapeutic relationship (Sinason, 2010; Simpson and Miller, 2004; Alvarez, 1992). This chapter will focus on groupwork with children whose disabilities significantly impact on their 'being in the world' because of the additional physical or sensory difficulties that can occur alongside intellectual disability, especially in the severe to profound range.

First, the notion of disability will be briefly explored in order to contextualize the different elements that need to be considered when working psychotherapeutically with children who have disabilities. Second, a general overview of interventions from group therapeutic play to psychotherapy through play will be discussed. This will be followed by a neuro-developmental approach to the building of relationships, providing the interpersonal framework for all therapeutic interventions. The earliest form of relationship will be explored where the child is helped to create a sense of self through playful interaction. The fostering of social connection, the awareness of the other, will then be considered through the use of groupwork that uses an embodied approach with the focus on rhythm, music and movement. Finally, practical considerations in setting up and running groups for children with disabilities will be discussed.

Understanding disability

Living with a disability in contemporary, western society inherently means living within a system that discriminates against, and excludes to varying degrees, all those whose bodies and minds do not fit within the accepted notion of normative functioning (Wendell, 1996; Garland Thomson, 2009; Snyder and Mitchell, 2006; Linton, 2007; Goodley *et al.* 2012). This is the lived reality of disability. What should be experienced as a shared interdependence, and an acceptance of vulnerability between all members of a community, often becomes a disempowering experience with disability being perceived as deficit and loss, rather than an alternative way of being.

Having witnessed such disempowerment time and time again as a member of a multidisciplinary clinical team working with children and adults with disabilities, it became obvious that the communal response to those who are differently abled tends to be based on a combination of not only pity, but also at times an underlying fear and need for avoidance. This can be a reflexive reaction related to a primordial emotional response that identifies difference as threatening (Cozolino, 2006, p. 266). When disability is considered as a social construction, it uncovers the existence of negating learned responses that are expressed as an uncomfortable sympathy coupled with a patronizing admiration for the disabled individual, imagining an ongoing struggle for survival as a result of the burden of being disabled. Sometimes an even greater degree of admiration is extended to the perceived 'carers' of those with disabilities, reflecting an understanding of disability that is based on deficit and rehabilitation, an inherently medical interpretation of embodied difference as 'abnormal' (Longmore, 2009, p. 143). It is not an uncommon occurrence for well-intentioned but thoroughly misguided comments to be made, oblivious to the presence of the disabled child or adult, such as 'Ah, the poor thing, at least he doesn't know how bad he is …', 'Aren't you wonderful, doing this kind of work', 'What's wrong with him, was he born like that?' The non-disabled professionals involved in the care of disabled clients can easily be drawn into accepting a societally imposed regulatory role, containing their clients either within a regime of attempted normalization and acquiescence (Sinason, 2010, p. 23), or upholding an exclusionary, ableist understanding of disability as 'not really-human' (Kumari Campbell, 2012, p. 215). Play therapy offers one means of redressing this imbalance, providing an experience of relationship that focuses on the person, not the disability. This is what makes play therapy such an effective intervention for disabled children, even those with severe to profound intellectual disabilities. For any therapist working in this field, personal preconceived notions of disability need to be explored and challenged so that therapeutic relationships can be formed that are fully open to the humanity of the other.

The continuum of play and therapeutic intervention

Playing is a fundamental aspect of life. Through play, experience is assimilated, possibilities are explored and inner subjectivity meets with outer reality in play's creative expression of 'being in the world'. Neuroscientist Jaak Panksepp (2009) includes play as one of the seven innate emotional systems, with early play being essential for the growth of social interaction. For a child with multiple disabilities, play often requires the support of another person; it cannot always happen with the level of spontaneity that other children experience. As the child's needs are multiple and complex, there is the danger that play becomes a functional means of meeting targets set in other clinical interventions such as speech and language therapy, physiotherapy or occupational therapy. Consequently, the emphasis can often be placed on teaching rather than on simply playing. It is vital that a balance is achieved so that the child is provided with as many play experiences as possible outside these constraints, along the whole continuum of playful activity.

Through the facilitation of play within the therapeutic relationship, the play therapist is offering a means of communication that isn't dependent on the child's linguistic skills or even on the child's ability to make use of toys as such. Playful interaction occurs from birth and doesn't require a particular threshold of cognitive functioning; it is rooted in the interpersonal connection that is engendered within each interaction (Trevarthen, 2003).

In the play room, the child is met in his way of being, at that particular moment in time. By engaging a child through the medium of play, an intersubjective relationship can be built where the child is given the experience of empathic attunement, which allows for growth and change to occur (Schore, 2009; Cozolino, 2006; Landreth, 2001). When this playful interaction occurs at the developmental level that is appropriate to the individual child in the therapeutic play session, it is of benefit along a continuum of needs. For children with intellectual disabilities, this can cover a range of objectives. Where multiple disabilities are present, there is often a negative impact on the child's play development, as opportunities for early exploratory play and interactions with the child's environment will probably have been severely limited. There is a tendency for such children to become passive onlookers, experiencing play by proxy, rather than by active engagement. Where this is the case, the child's play repertoire can be extended by the therapist through the use of adapted toys and 'hand over hand' facilitation. In the initial sessions, it is often necessary to be quite directive and to introduce play sequences to the child so that the potential for exploration, communication and expression contained within the play room can be fully accessed and realized. Toys have to be introduced and, through guided exploration, the child becomes aware of possible uses and discovers ways of successfully interacting physically with objects, allowing play to become more complex. This can be embedded in a structured therapeutic group play session where a shared theme, such as a simple story, can be adapted to include sensory play in order to provide an embodied experience of the story's narrative.

A child with an intellectual disability will often benefit from having his or her play scaffolded at times in order to fully develop the child's potential to use the play therapeutically. This is an element that is often built in to the natural flow of a client centred group session, where the therapist makes a suggestion which will expand the play without interfering with the child's intent at the time. This is not a didactic approach as the child is free to engage with the suggestion or ignore it, without fear of disapproval or any sense of failure. When new ideas are introduced with sensitivity in this way, the child will often embrace the suggestion and incorporate the new idea into his own play.

The social aspects of therapeutic group play introduce the basic notions of turn taking and sharing, empowerment and self-esteem but the supportive role of the therapist needs to be more active and directive in order to counteract any limitations, particularly physical, created by the children's disabilities. Through focussed interventions, play skills can be developed and enhanced, and developmental gains may be attained. Paediatric occupational therapist and play therapist Karen Stagnitti's developmental play programme (1998) fosters imaginative play, and psychiatrist Stanley Greenspan's *Floortime* (1998) approach focuses on creating relationship and communication through directed play with children who have developmental delays, particularly those with Autistic Spectrum Disorder. Together, these approaches offer a comprehensive base to play expansion that will increase the play skills of children with disabilities. Sensory needs can be met in a therapeutic play setting, especially when the child is dependent on the assistance of others in order to interact with his environment. Such interventions are particularly suitable for group based sessions – for example, messy play programmes – where the child is physically facilitated to explore his environment at a developmentally appropriate level.

With a psychotherapeutic intent, playful interactions can be reparative, allowing the child to regain what has been lost or damaged through negative life experiences. For a child with a disability, this is particularly relevant as there is an increased likelihood of issues arising from such things as hospitalizations, emotional difficulties resulting from the social stigma often associated with disability and the day-to-day frustrations of living in a world that does not adequately meet the physical, social and emotional needs of the child (Hodges and Sheppard, 2004). The therapist needs to have a sensitive awareness of the impact that all these factors may have on the child's emotional wellbeing.

Working psychotherapeutically through play with disabled children requires a flexible approach, where the usual parameters and guidelines that govern play therapy often need to be considered in a more creative way. For example, making a simple choice to pick up a toy depends on the child's ability to scan the available objects, focus on one particular thing, reach out and pick up that object. For a child with disabilities, multiple factors may need to be considered. If the child has a difficulty with sensory processing, too many objects may be confusing and overwhelming, and choicemaking becomes almost impossible. For a child with cerebral palsy, co-ordinating gross and fine motor movements in order to reach out and grasp an object may be beyond that child's physical capacity. For a child with a visual impairment, other senses need to be facilitated in order to explore the available choices.

All of these possibilities involve the therapist taking a more pro-active role as facilitator, whether working with a child individually or within a group, so that the child is given the freedom to interact as fully as possible. Similarly, building a therapeutic relationship with a child who has multiple disabilities needs to be thought about in light of the child's developmental level, along with any physical or sensory difficulties. For the child to experience empathic attunement, the therapist must be extremely sensitive not only to the child's embodied presence, but also to her own. Verbal interaction may be severely limited, so all non-verbal means of communication become vitally important. Understanding these communications can be a frustrating process for both child and therapist and a great deal of patience is often required – along with a sense of humour!

Katie, a non-verbal child with cerebral palsy who used her eyes very eloquently to communicate a need, tried desperately to direct my attention downwards. She looked with great intensity at me, then at her feet. I followed her gaze and began to guess what she was trying to communicate. 'Is it your feet?' She thought for a moment and shook her head to indicate 'No!'; '...your shoes?', she looked a little more excited and indicated a more vehement 'Yes ... no!!'; '...do you want me to adjust the footplate of your wheelchair?' This elicited a very impatient and irritated 'No!!!' her face angry and her body arching with the intensity of her answer. She kept repeating her eye pointing with even more intensity as I tried to interpret her meaning. We were both becoming frustrated. I reflected this and how hard it was for us, her trying to tell, me not yet understanding, and sometimes getting it very, very wrong. I suggested that I try some wild guesses, a strategy we had used before where my more imaginative attempts often brought us to laughter. It not only reduced the growing frustration, but also sometimes threw up unexpected results. This was one of those times. I began to offer interpretations, and suggested that perhaps her real aim was to make me act like one of those 'nodding dogs' that bobs its head up and down continuously, looking at her, looking at her feet. She laughed uproariously at this suggestion and got very, very excited. Following the trail she was giving me by her embodied responses, a few more questions brought us to the important news she had been trying to share, her puppy had chewed a pair of her socks the previous day.

Katie's overt communications left me in no doubt as to whether or not I was on the right track in my attempts at understanding this glimpse of her life that she so eagerly wanted to share. It is not always as straightforward as the imparting of a story. Communicating wishes, desires, feeling states, or a myriad other messages can be fraught with difficulty for someone who has non-typical communication skills.

Dramatherapist Anna Chesner puts it very succinctly:

> Everyday social interaction depends on a complex web of signs and symbols, some of which the person with learning disabilities may not have learnt, or may not be physically capable of performing. It is only too easy to jump to wrong conclusions when interpreting what we see.
> (1995, p. 18)

This is why transference and counter-transference become essential tools for interpreting communications that cannot be spoken. This will be discussed now in more depth as part of the intersubjectivity that is present in the therapeutic relationship.

Building relationship: creating a sense of self through playful interaction

Before a child can successfully engage with others in a group situation, there first needs to be a sense of self within the intersubjectivity that is created when two people engage with each other. This engagement is at the core of the relationship between therapist and client and the child's non-verbal micro-communications are the building blocks of this relationship. Once they are established, the child can then begin to relate to others in the group. Developing a sense of self has its roots in the first experience of relating that occurs between an infant and the primary care giver, where moments of synchrony come about (Hughes, 2007). Recent neurobiological developments are uncovering the essentially social aspects of the human brain, demonstrating how we are 'hardwired' to seek interaction with others (Siegel, 2012;

Schore, 2012). Developmental psychologist Colwyn Trevarthen's research with new-born infants has shown that a baby as young as twenty minutes old will interact with an adult, 'demonstrating coherence of its intentionality and its awareness of a world outside the body, and especially a world that offers live company' (2003, p. 57). It is this level of interaction that needs to be awakened within the therapeutic setting, providing the basis for growth and change. For children with severe to profound intellectual disabilities, these pre-verbal patterns of interaction need to be gradually developed in a one-to-one therapeutic situation so that an experience of successful relationship is created that can then be built upon. Sensorimotor psychotherapist Pat Ogden describes this process:

> The therapist meticulously watches for incipient spontaneous actions and affects – the beginnings of a smile, meaningful eye contact, a more expansive and playful movement – that indicate positive affect, and capitalizes on those moments by participating in kind and/or calling attention to them and expressing curiosity, enabling the moment to linger ... and help expand their regulatory boundaries.
>
> (2009, p. 221)

Building this relationship can be a very slow process and some children would be overwhelmed if placed in a group setting before their ability to emotionally regulate had not first matured sufficiently.

Jodie, a seven-year-old girl with severe intellectual disability, was brought to the playroom by a carer who spoke brightly to her as she steered Jodie's wheelchair towards the door. Jodie was holding her hands in front of her face and rocking her body, making a high pitched keening noise as the carer left and the door shut behind her. Slowly, I approached Jodie and sat near her, quietly singing the low pitched, gentle 'hello' song that signified the start of our session together. I watched carefully for signs that Jodie's hyper-aroused state was beginning to decrease. Her rocking began to match the rhythm of the song and her keening began to decrease in volume. The song ended, I paused for a few moments and then asked, 'Again?' Jodie stilled, peeped from between her fingers, and grunted. This time, we sang together as Jodie's keening took on a different quality, joining with me as we both rocked rhythmically and a smile of recognition began to spread slowly across her face. The song ended and I offered my hand, reaching out without actually making direct contact. Her rocking slowed, stopped, and hesitantly Jodie touched my hand briefly with hers, suddenly withdrawing but no longer covering her face with her hands. We repeated this interaction several times while I spoke in the 'motherese' (Trevarthen, 2009) tones similar to the interactions of a primary care giver with a young infant. A turn taking pattern developed, with me leaving space for Jodie to respond to my vocalizations with both her voice and her actions, as she began to instigate the touching together of our hands. Jodie's breathing rate began to increase, her rocking began again and one hand reached up to her face. This was the signal for me to withdraw as Jodie was beginning to become hyper-aroused again and needed quiet time in which to regain homeostasis and assimilate our interaction. After several minutes, Jodie was again ready to engage with me.

We repeated this pattern several times before the session ended. Slowly, over a period of months, Jodie was able to tolerate longer periods of interaction, which became more complex and with increased playfulness as we shared games of 'peekaboo', sang and danced together and began to join together in sensory play. Jodie began to explore the playroom with my facilitation, showing interest and developing shared attention in the toys and activities I offered. Her increased ability to regulate her affective states had matured enough so that she was now ready to join in group sessions.

Allan Schore's research into affect regulation in infants is particularly relevant to therapeutic work in the field of intellectual disability. He has shown that the change mechanism is not necessarily mediated by insight, but is the product of an experience of therapeutic synchrony. He states that 'psychotherapy is not the "talking cure" but the affect communicating and regulating cure' (2009, p. 128). In the transference and counter-transference between child and therapist, affects are communicated through right brain emotional relational processes, not through language. This could clearly be seen in the interactions with Jodie. Schore goes on to explain that in order to know about the client's unconscious process, we need to become not only keen observers of our clients' physiology and the associated bodily changes – such as body position, facial expression, shifts in eye gaze, changes in muscle tension and breathing – but also fully aware of our own physiological responses and what they are communicating, as well as the emotional content of our presence.

In the dance of communication, therapist and child can achieve synchrony through a pattern of engagement, arousal, withdrawal and re-engagement. This replicates the early pattern of rupture and repair (Schore, 1994) where infants learn to differentiate and separate from their mothers, develop self-regulation, tolerate waiting and frustration and develop further interactional skills. In therapy, children with severe intellectual disabilities tend to be at this level of interaction and the therapeutic relationship gives the opportunity for the child to experience synchrony with another. Where symbolic play is absent and communication is non-verbal, relatedness becomes more important than cognition (Corbett, 2009) and interpretation can be communicated in a way that is receivable – it can be 'held' in the therapist's mind rather than verbalized. The therapist becomes a thinking presence on behalf of the child and gives meaning to interactions through her embodied self and her use of voice. The pitch, timbre and rhythm of her vocalizations can 'provide an aural sense of holding and containment' (ibid. 2009, p. 49).

Underlying all of this is the ongoing creation of a shared language, the fundamental work that starts with the therapist being attentive to every nuance of the child's presence in the room and offering responses that acknowledge these communications, opening the door for more complex and meaningful interactions. This is often a slow process that demands patience from both the child and the therapist as each searches for the other's meaning and intent.

At the beginning of our therapeutic relationship, David used tapping in attempting to regulate himself whenever he began to experience emotional overwhelm. As a non-verbal eleven-year-old with a dual diagnosis of severe intellectual disability and Autistic Spectrum Disorder, he liked predictability and calm. Unexpected occurrences upset him and he had created a means of calming himself. He tapped with his fingertips on any available surface, doors, windows, walls or tables; if holding an object in his hand, that became a tool for tapping. He would become completely absorbed in his actions, oblivious to his surroundings in his need to self-soothe. Whenever it occurred, I began to match his tapping in the pauses, mirroring the intensity of his actions with my own and using my words and voice to reflect the quality of his emotional state. Each time I vocalized, I gradually modulated my voice and actions, supporting David with this external regulatory mechanism to help him regain a sense of calm, as you would with a very young infant. He responded well to my joining in and together we usually managed to reduce the intensity of his anxiety. David became curious. He began to tap when not anxious, watching for my response and smiling when I replicated the rhythmic pattern of his taps. Over time, a game developed between us as he varied his rhythms and extended the tapping to include different surfaces. I introduced drumsticks and a drum, David included shakers and a tambourine. The volume began to vary, along with the length and complexity of the rhythms as we alternated leading and following. The game invariably ended with a crescendo of noise as we both gleefully tapped and bashed our rhythms simultaneously. What had begun as a regulatory behaviour had evolved into having several shared meanings and purposes for David. He further extended this use of sound and rhythm to actively express his emotional states, seeking an empathic, attuned response through his actions. In a sad moment, for example, his taps were slow and lethargic. When I mirrored his sadness both verbally and in my tapping response, tears welled in his eyes and we shared the depth of his communicated feeling.

Attuned mirroring of his actions had provided David with an entry point into an interpersonal communication from a position of isolation. His increased tolerance of novelty and spontaneity in his individual sessions made it possible to include him in a therapeutic group that focussed on the use of music to build social interaction. David was able to cope with this more challenging environment and to engage with social interactions within the group.

By mirroring David's actions along with the emotional content of his embodied communication, an interpersonal connection was made at the most fundamental level. Psychiatrist and neuroscientist Daniel Siegel speaks of the mirror neuron system in the brain that allows us to connect in this way with others' minds. Siegel states:

> We use our first five senses to take in the signals from another person. Then the mirror neuron system perceives these 'intentional states', and by way of the insula alters the limbic and body states to match those we are seeing in the other person. This is attunement and it creates emotional resonance.
>
> (2007, p. 167)

Through the dynamic relationship between child and therapist, with playful interaction as the primary means of communication, complex social and emotional issues can be addressed in a clinically safe, contained and effective way. The child is met at his or her developmental level through the therapist's sensitivity to his mode of communication, valuing both embodied and projective expression of inner subjectivity, and so making therapeutic change possible. For David, his limitations in verbal communication and cognitive ability did not prevent him from engaging in the therapeutic process. Psychotherapist Jason Upton states:

> despite any challenges of poor memory, poor verbal and communication skills, or poor capacity for cognitive linking, clients can still express their life experiences, their perceptions and understanding, and their emotional and behavioural responses to life. These are the fundamental prerequisites for the therapeutic process to take place.
>
> (2009, pp. 33–34)

Building a relationship with an empathically attuned therapist allows this to happen. It also creates the possibility for the building of other relationships that can meet social and emotional needs outside the therapy space. Groupwork supports the development of other relationships in a safe and contained way, creating a social microcosm of acceptance and support.

Making connections: interpersonal relationships in groups

Where group participants have intellectual disabilities, the most effective means of fostering relationships is through activities that rely on embodied expressions of 'being in the world', such as dance and movement. The use of rhythmic sound and movement in the therapy session can mirror the early experience of the predictable maternal rhythms of early life, which form the basis of trust (Trevarthen, 2003).

At a prenatal level, a synchronicity is already being created between mother and foetus through the shared experience of biological and physical rhythms. The mother's heartbeat, breathing, the bodily actions of everyday life such as walking and the act of speech, all provide an interweaving of rhythm and movement that shape early experience. The intrauterine environment of auditory, vibratory, proprioceptive and kinaesthetic stimuli provides the earliest form of attunement (Maiello, 2001).

At a somatic level, this attunement continues to develop postnatally through the physical holding, which provides the continuation of shared rhythms already experienced, and the use of 'motherese', those singsong vocalisations of mother to infant that are found globally (Schore, 2012; Schwartz *et al.* 2003; Schogler and Trevarthen, 2007). The tone of voice used, the pitch and the variation all create a deep connection with the infant and are a vital element of the bonding process. The use of songs and nursery rhymes can replicate this early experience. The verbal content is very much secondary, it is the rhythm that is communicated that reflects the beat/pause, beat/pause link with the presence/absence of the mother, as the delicate dance of interpersonal relationship is being formed. These are the fundamental aspects of the development of relationship that can be supported in group settings. Psychotherapist Suzanne Maiello has examined the presence of rhythm in enabling the brain to form relationships. She states:

> There exists a connection between rhythmicity of maternal embodiment providing the music of the life dance, and the holding of the infant in early attachment/ attunement patterns, where mirror neurons are creating the groundwork for the development of empathy through rhythmic sound and movement. It seems that rhythmical qualities of the earliest interpersonal experiences become part of a deeply rooted knowledge of how to relate to other human beings.
>
> (2001, p. 181)

Dance is a non-judgemental medium with no right or wrong way to move. Each individual is free to move in a way that reflects conscious and unconscious thoughts and feelings. For a person with no verbal communication, movement can become a way of developing a relationship that is a support in his personal journey, as well as a means by which the therapist can witness the expression of his inner life. In this way, it can be a conversation between participants, acknowledging each person's presence as an individual with autonomy and agency. For someone with a profound intellectual disability, rhythmic movement provides a link that makes the outside world accessible where otherwise there is isolation and can be the first step in moving towards an emerging sense of self (Maiello, 2001, p. 182). Dance activities can create an experience of inter-relationship where there is a shared acceptance of each other's presence. For children who often experience life as 'outsiders', being part of a group and engaging in a communal activity within the containment of therapeutic space can give a sense of acceptance that affirms each child's self-worth.

Practical considerations when working with groups

There are many diverse factors that need to be taken into account when setting up and running a group for children with disabilities and it can be a rather complicated process with the therapist acting almost as a detective when considering the inclusion of a child in a particular group. It is helpful to observe the child in advance, in different settings, in order to gain as comprehensive an understanding of the child's needs as possible. Information can be gathered from family members, carers and other professionals, and perhaps particular medical conditions and syndromes might need to be researched in order to inform therapy decisions. Working with a child with a disability also means working with those who are part of that child's life. This brings about its own potential benefits and disadvantages: those that know the child well can provide invaluable information such as the child's methods of communication, or their emotional states and how they are expressed; on the other hand, if those involved in the child's care are not understanding of, and committed to, the process of therapy, this can have a very negative effect on the child's experience and the therapy can be undermined (Cottis and O'Driscoll, 2009).

Pre-therapy considerations need to be carefully thought about regarding the availability of ongoing emotional support between sessions, along with such mundane things as ensuring that the child can be brought to the sessions on a regular basis. All the attendant details regarding physical support and care during therapy sessions for a child with a high level of needs have to be considered. Running a play therapy group for children with multiple disabilities requires a higher level of planning and more dependence on others for assistance in order to ensure that the group can be run successfully.

Along with the usual factors when formulating a plan for group play therapy sessions, there are some practical considerations that need to be kept in mind when working with children with disabilities. This is by no means a comprehensive list, but a highlighting of some basic elements.

Creating the group

Group members need to be chosen carefully, matching their developmental needs and personal preferences as closely as possible. For example, a child with auditory sensitivity should not be placed into a group of children where the noise level may become unbearable. Clear guidelines are needed for any other adults present as to their level of involvement, so that they know what is expected of them. The number of adults necessary to support and facilitate activities (for example, sensory and messy play sessions) where a therapeutic play approach is being used, needs to be carefully considered. In school settings, Special Needs Assistants can often be available to help with 'hand over hand' activities, enabling the child to interact with his environment. It is the therapist's responsibility to ensure that the child's communications are being recognized and responded to appropriately. This will avoid the potential difficulty of facilitation becoming too directive and didactic, thus reducing the child's autonomy and sense of empowerment.

Structuring the session

A clear start and end is needed for each session. For a child with an intellectual disability, transitions from one activity to another can be difficult enough, so the transition from one way of being to another when entering and leaving the therapy session needs to be very sensitively managed by the therapist. The intense experience of empathic attunement within the therapeutic alliance needs to be clearly boundaried and contained within the therapy session, both psychically and physically, with the room and the therapist remaining a secure base. A variety of strategies can be used to ensure this happens. Depending on the children's developmental level, it can be a very concrete ritual such as taking shoes off at the beginning and having them put back on at the end of the session. A specific song is often sung that would not be heard elsewhere in the children's daily lives, and this is used to greet or say goodbye to each child, acknowledging their presence within the group. A particular section of the room may be the starting point for a movement game.

Whatever the ritual, it is important that it remains constant every session, repeating exactly the same sequence so that continuity and predictability are established. This also fosters the sense of belonging that is a fundamental aspect of group work, especially in the field of disability.

The use of observation and repetition

The more severe the intellectual disability, the greater the need for observation and repetition. There is no substitute for close observation. Through noticing even the most subtle changes in each child's embodied presence, a knowledge bank can be built up regarding that child's communications, creating the foundations for empathic attunement. Repetition of interactions, communications and shared activities can attach meaning to what otherwise might be perceived by the child as random occurrences. By the use of repetition within each session, even children with profound intellectual disabilities can begin to recognize and anticipate the sequence of activities, enhancing the experience of being part of a group. The same sequence of activities throughout a series of sessions can provide a sense of familiarity that not only offers security, but also of competence and empowerment.

Conclusion

Through group play therapy for children with disabilities, interpersonal connection can be created and developed where otherwise there might have been isolation, play skills can be expanded and facilitated and emotional needs can be met within a social context.

When all essential factors are considered and necessary arrangements are put in place, the group itself can offer an incredibly rich experience for both the clients and the therapist. Building relationships in a therapeutic setting holds the potential to have a transformative effect on the lives of participants where each is met fully as a person, not as a collection of symptoms, behaviours that need adapting or difficulties that need treatment.

Key points

1. For children with multiple disabilities, play therapy acknowledges the presence of an active emotional life and nurtures the child's capacity to engage in a therapeutic relationship.

2. The therapist engages with the child at a non-verbal, embodied level that reflects early attachment patterns based on synchrony, affect regulation and empathic attunement.
3. Play therapy practice often has to be adapted to facilitate actions and interactions, and to provide experiential opportunities for children who cannot easily access their environment. For children with severe disabilities, embodied practice including dance, movement and rhythm creates a shared, non-verbal means of communication.

References

Alvarez, A. (1992). *Live Company. Psychoanalytic Therapy with Autistic, Borderline, Deprived and Abused Children.* London: Routledge.

Chesner, A. (1995). *Dramatherapy for People with Learning Disabilities.* London: Jessica Kingsley.

Corbett, A. (2009). Words as a second language: The psychotherapeutic challenge of severe intellectual disability. In T. Cottis (ed.), *Intellectual Disability, Trauma and Psychotherapy.* New York: Routledge.

Cottis, T. and O'Driscoll, D. (2009). Outside in: The effects of trauma on organizations. In T. Cottis (ed.), *Intellectual Disability, Trauma and Psychotherapy.* New York: Routledge.

Cozolino, L. (2006). *The Neuroscience of Human Relationships.* New York: Norton.

Fosha, D., Siegel, D. and Solomon, M. (eds) (2009). *The Healing Power of Emotion.* New York: Norton.

Garland Thomson, R. (2009). *Staring: How We Look.* New York: Oxford University Press.

Goodley, D., Hughes, B. and Davis, L. (eds) (2012). *Disability and Social Theory. New Developments and Directions.* New York: Palgrave Macmillan.

Greenspan, S. and Weider, S. (1998). *The Child with Special Needs.* Cambridge MA: DaCapo Press.

Hodges, S. and Sheppard, N. (2004). Therapeutic dilemmas when working with a group of children with physical and learning disabilities. In D. Simpson and L. Miller (eds) *Unexpected Gains. Psychotherapy with People with Learning Disabilities.* London: Karnac.

Hughes, D. (2007). *Attachment Focused Family Therapy.* New York: Norton.

Kumari Campbell, F. (2012). Stalking ableism: Using disability to expose 'abled' narcissism. In D. Goodley, B. Hughes and L. Davis (eds) *Disability and Social Theory: New Developments and Directions.* Basingstoke: Palgrave Macmillan.

Landreth, G. (2001). Facilitative dimensions of play in the play therapy process. In G. Landreth (ed.) *Innovations in Play Therapy. Issues, Processes and Special Populations.* New York: Brunner Routledge.

Linton, S. (2007). *My Body Politic.* Ann Arbor: University of Michigan Press.

Longmore, P. (2009). The second phase: From disability rights to disability culture. In R. Baird, S. Rosenbaum, S. Kay Tombs (eds) *Disability: The Social, Political and Ethical Debate*. New York: Prometheus Books.

Maiello, S. (2001). On temporal shapes: The relation between primary rhythmical experience and the quality of mental links. In J. Edwards (ed.) *Being Alive: Building on the Work of Anne Alvarez*. Hove: Brunner Routledge.

Malloch, S. and Trevarthen, C. (eds) (2009). *Communicative Musicality: Exploring the Basis of Human Companionship*. Oxford: Oxford University Press.

Ogden, P. (2009). Emotion, mindfulness and movement: Expanding the regulatory boundaries of the window of affect tolerance. In D. Fosha, D. Siegel and M. Solomon (eds) *The Healing Power of Emotion*. New York: Norton.

Panksepp, J. (2009). The emotional antecedents to the evolution of music and language. *Musicae Scientae* 13 (2), 229–259.

Schogler, B. and Trevarthen, C. (2007). To sing and dance together: From infants to jazz. In S. Bråten (ed) *On Being Moved: From Mirror Neurons to Empathy*. Amsterdam: John Benjamins.

Schore, A. (2009). Right brain affect regulation. In D. Fosha, D. Siegel and M. Solomon (eds) *The Healing Power of Emotion. Affective Neuroscience, Development and Clinical Practice*. New York: Norton.

— (2012). *The Science of the Art of Psychotherapy*. New York: Norton.

— (2001). Neurobiology, developmental psychology, and psychoanalysis. Convergent findings on the subject of projective identification. In J. Edwards (ed.) *Being Alive*. New York: Taylor and Francis.

— (1994). *Affect Regulation and the Origin of the Self: the Neurobiology of Emotional Development*. Hillsdale, NJ: Erlbaum.

Schwartz, D., Howe, C. Q. and Purves, D. (2003). The statistical structure of human speech sounds predicts musical universals. *Journal of Neuroscience* 23, 7160–7168.

Siegel, D. (2012). *The Developing Mind: How Relationships and the Brain Interact to Shape Who We Are* (2nd edn). New York: Guilford Press.

Simpson, D. and Miller, L. (eds) (2004). *Unexpected Gains: Psychotherapy with People with Learning Disabilities*. London: Karnac.

Sinason, V. (2010). *Mental Handicap and the Human Condition* (2nd edn). London: Free Association Books.

Snyder, S. and Mitchell, D. (2006). Afterword – Regulated bodies: Disability studies and the controlling professions. In D. Turner and K. Stagg (eds) *Disability and Deformity*. Oxford: Routledge.

Stagnitti, K. (1998). *Learn to Play*. Melbourne: Co-ordinates Publishers.

Trevarthen, C. (2003). Neuroscience and intrinsic dynamics: Current knowledge and potential for therapy. In J. Corrigal and H. Wilkinson (eds) *Revolutionary Connections: Psychotherapy and Neuroscience*. London: Karnac.

— (2009). The functions of emotion in infancy: The regulation and communication of rhythm, sympathy and meaning in human development. In D. Fosha, D. Siegel and M. Solomon (eds) *The Healing Power of Emotion*. New York: Norton.

Upton, J. (2009). When words are not enough: Creative therapeutic approaches. In T. Cottis (ed.) *Intellectual Disability, Trauma and Psychotherapy*. New York: Routledge.

Wendell, S. (1996). *The Rejected Body*. New York: Routledge.

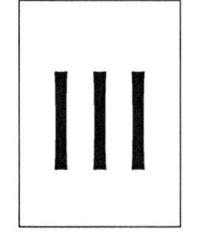

III Using play therapeutically with parents and carers

9

The *Parent Learn to Play* program

Building relationships through play

Karen Stagnitti

In a local weekend newspaper magazine, an article titled 'A different kind of miracle' (Wheatley, 2013) told the story of the stress and anguish of a family where the parents and grandparents were coming to terms with twins born with a rare condition which affected their ability to speak and move. After much emotional turmoil and searching the world for a diagnosis (which was successful) and a cure (which was not successful), the article finished with a quote by the maternal grandfather that his daughter's object was now to make a happy home. A happy home includes laughter and enjoyment of each other's company. It means that a parent sees their child for the person and not the diagnosis. For a parent who has a child with a diagnosis or difficulties in development, this journey is a harrowing journey as was the case in the family featured in the newspaper magazine. This chapter is about the *Parent Learn to Play* program. The aim of the *Parent Learn to Play* program is to build a parent's understanding of the play of their child and teach them how to interact with their child through play. It was developed for parents who have a child with developmental difficulties. The importance of the parent-child relationship is discussed below before the program is described.

The parent-child relationship

A parent's relationship with their child is fundamental to their child's development and emotional-social well-being. Sunderland (2007) and Norrie McCain *et al.* (2007) emphasise that the parent-child relationship shapes a young child's brain and influences their emotional life on a long-term basis. How connections within the brain are formed and unformed is influenced by experiences. In the first five years of life these experiences are largely within the child's family. In a parent-child relationship where there is warm and genuine care and love, hormones such as opioids and oxytocin are in dominance in the child's brain and these hormones bring feelings of being safe in a world full of comfort, wonder and interest (Sunderland, 2007). When parent-child interaction is one of abuse, non-care and little warmth, cortisol, adrenaline and noradrenaline are activated more often in the child's brain, making that child's world one of stress and threat (Sunderland, 2007).

Parents who provide warmth and care to their child tend to provide a rich environment which includes providing their child with places to explore and imaginative and creative play materials (Sunderland, 2007). Play, which Sunderland (2007) aligns with curiosity, exploration and a motivation to learn, is connected with many chemicals, especially dopamine, which is associated with directed purpose and energy. When dopamine and opioids are stimulated in combination, joy occurs (Sunderland, 2007). As a parent engages with their child in a warm and loving relationship and provides a rich environment to play, their child experiences joy, warmth and feelings of being safe and wanting to explore and be curious. This engagement in play between a parent and a child is most effective if the parent follows the child's lead in child-led play (Sunderland, 2007). Such a relationship is often explained in terms of secure attachment.

Attachment

Secure attachment is displayed by a child when they move towards a protective figure (such as a loving parent) in times of stress, and in non-stress times are happy to explore away from their parent. Our understanding of attachment is underpinned by the research of Bowlby (1982) and Ainsworth *et al.* (1978). Ainsworth *et al.* identified parental sensitivity as one of the factors of attachment that van IJzendoorn *et al.* (2007) interpreted as 'the parents' ability to perceive and interpret their children's attachment signals accurately and to be able and willing to respond promptly and adequately to those signals' (p. 598). Van IJzendoorn *et al.* (2007) explored parental sensitivity and attachment with 40 parents who had a child with difficulties in their development and 15 parents who had a typically developing child. They found that 48 per cent of the children with autism spectrum disorder (ASD) showed secure attachment when presented with Ainsworth *et al.*'s (1978) Strange Situation procedure, but they also showed the highest percentage of children with disorganised attachment. To gather information on parental sensitivity and child involvement, van IJzendoorn *et al.* observed parents in a ten minute, free play situation with their child. Parents who had a child with ASD were not significantly different in parental sensitivity to parents who had a child without ASD. The predicted association between higher parental sensitivity with higher attachment security was not found with parents with children with ASD. Instead, higher parental sensitivity was associated with lower attachment security by the child. The children with ASD showed more disorganised and less involvement with their parents than children without ASD (van IJzendoorn *et al.* 2007). Van IJzendoorn *et al.* (2007) put forward that their study tested the limits of attachment theory, particularly for children with ASD, as attachment security manifested itself differently. They suggested that proximity-seeking and contact-maintaining may have a different function for these children.

Attachment is often measured through a child's play with dolls or through observations of the quality of free play between the parent and the child (e.g. Green *et al.* 2000; van IJzendoorn *et al.* 2007). The connection between play and attachment is summed up by Naber *et al.* (2008): 'Children with secure attachment relationships display more sophisticated, complex and diverse play during interactions with their mother and during solitary play' (p. 858). Naber *et al.* (2008) explored play behaviour and attachment in children with ASD and found that children with ASD with a secure attachment had higher levels of play and spent more time playing. They interpreted their findings as evidence that a secure attachment with the parent contributed to better play outcomes for children with ASD. Naber *et al.* (2008) suggested that interventions which focussed on improving play ability should also focus 'on enhancing the quality of the attachment relationship' (p. 864).

This chapter outlines the *Parent Learn to Play* program, which was developed to build a parent's understanding of their child's play and how to interact with their child through play. As the program is aimed at parents who have a child with a developmental difficulty, it is a secondary aim of the program that the child and parent relationship would become closer. Much of the work with parents and children through the *Parent Learn to Play* program has been with parents who have a child with ASD, so this chapter concentrates on these parents and children. A search of other parent programs found programs that instructed parents on how to manage their child's behaviour. No programs were located where play between a parent and a child was the complete focus.

Theoretical underpinnings of the *Parent Learn to Play* program

The *Parent Learn to Play* program is strongly influenced by child-centred play therapy as outlined by Axline (1974), together with the cognitive developmental theories of play, particularly those of Lev Vygotsky. Axline (1974) was a student of Carl Rogers and developed her work with children from his foundational work in person-centred therapy. An adaption of Axline's eight principles is fundamental to the approach of the therapist when demonstrating how to engage a child in play with the parent. These are: the therapist develops a warm relationship with the child; the therapist accepts the child unconditionally; the therapist creates an atmosphere of permissiveness so the child is free to self-initiate; the therapist respects the parent and child's capacity to develop; the child leads the way and therapy follows the pace of the child; the therapist responds to the child; the only limits established are those that allow the play to flow. In contrast to Axline's approach, praising is used to encourage the child to repeat a play skill. Praise is used in a focussed way to direct the child's attention to what they are playing and to encourage the child to continue while, at the same time, accepting any change the child may make to the play direction.

The value of play to child development and the play skills in the *Parent Learn to Play* program are informed by the cognitive developmental theories of play. Cognitive developmental theorists assume that play involves the use of symbols and that play is distinguished from other general forms of activity by the creation of imaginary situations (see Vygotsky, 1966). Play behaviour is synonymous with the attribute of pretending in play and pretend play is understood to be a leading factor in child development (Vygotsky, 1966).

Vygotsky (1997) emphasized a sociocultural dimension to play and cognition and placed emphasis on the social context of the child. He explained how the 'zone of proximal development' increased children's actual development to their potential development through adult guidance and more experienced peers (Vygotsky, 1997). Vygotsky (1997) considered that children's cognitive development varied according to social activity and the language of a more competent other. Hence, enhancing how a parent plays with their child who has a developmental difficulty should enrich their child's social context and development.

The focus of the *Parent Learn to Play* is on pretend play because pretend play (also called imaginative play, make-believe play, representational play or fantasy play) is the quintessence of play (Stagnitti, 2004). Pretend play is a unique type of play because children impose meaning on a situation, they substitute one object for another (e.g. a box for a bed), they attribute properties to objects and actions (e.g. the doll is hungry or the car is fast), and they refer to absent objects (e.g. money is exchanged by the movement of the hand in the pocket and then moving the hand to meet the hand of another). There is limited research on pretend play and the brain but the research that has been published has shown that many areas of the brain light up when adults watch pretend play. These include those areas for theory of mind and emotional gestures

(Whitehead *et al.* 2009), narrative (German *et al.* 2004; Whitehead *et al.* 2009), language comprehension (Whitehead *et al.* 2009) and frontal areas of the brain involved in controlling strong emotions, planning, reflecting, thinking about emotional experiences and being sensitive to others' emotional and social cues (Sunderland, 2007; German *et al.* 2004; Whitebread *et al.* 2009).

The *Parent Learn to Play* program

The *Parent Learn to Play* program grew out of the *Learn to Play* program (Stagnitti, 1998). *Learn to Play* aims to build the spontaneous ability of a child to self-initiate their own play. For children to benefit from the program they need to have reached 12 to 18 months developmental level and have one meaningful word or gesture. *Learn to Play* grew out of my clinical work with children in early childhood intervention. Years before, I had been working with children using child-centred play therapy (Axline, 1974). While I loved this work, I came to realise that one of Axline's assumptions was that children know how to play. As I started to understand play in more depth and measure a child's ability to play, I became aware that many of the children I was working with in early childhood intervention did not know how to play. *Learn to Play* grew out of a realization that a program was needed to show children how to play. From this program has grown the *Parent Learn to Play* program.

The *Parent Learn to Play* program shows parents how to engage with their child in pretend play and how to respond to their child in play to encourage the child to self-initiate and extend their play. Much of the work to date has been with parents who have a child with autism or an intellectual disability and I will concentrate on these parent-child dyads as I explain the program. The *Parent Learn to Play* program is composed of a Foundation program and an Intermediate program. The Advanced program is when the parent runs all the sessions. The program takes parents through 12 skills that children require in order to pretend in play. Each skill builds on the next. By the end of the program, parents have commented that they had not appreciated that play was such a complex ability. The program can be run in one of three ways. One way is with a large group of parents over six hours of training, divided into two three-hour sessions. In these sessions the parents are taken through the skills of play and given time to practise the skill with their partner or other parents in small groups. Another way is to spread the sessions over 12 one-hour sessions where small groups of parents are taken through each skill and more time is given to practice and discussion of how to engage their own child. The other way is in parent-child dyads. In this approach, the child's play ability is assessed as this gives guidance to where the program begins. The 12 skills are then spread over 24 weeks in 12 fortnightly blocks. In the first week of a fortnight block, the therapist models the skill by engaging with the child in play and in the second week the parent runs the session with their child, with the therapist facilitating the session. This chapter will concentrate on this latter approach to the program.

The 12 skills of the program take the parent through each new play skill while building on the previous skill. In reality, because play is so complex, several play skills will be included in each session. For example, 'having cups of tea with teddy' could include the skills of play script (domestic theme); sequences of play action (for example, pouring the tea (first action), putting cup to lips (second action), stirring the cup (third action), putting cup to lips (fourth action)); decentration (the teddy is 'alive' and is drinking); and describing the play. However, as a therapist you understand this and are monitoring this throughout the session so that the child remains engaged with the play, but to the parent you are demonstrating just one skill and showing the parent what this looks like in play with their child. For example, you may only be concentrating on 'sequences of play action' and so you point out to the parent the actions their child is able to undertake spontaneously and with imitation. A summary of the content of the program is given in Table 9.1. The play skills listed in Table 9.1 are either missing or poorly executed in the play of children with ASD. It is not uncommon for children to enter the program with no or little play ability.

Table 9.1 Content and underpinning skills of the *Parent Learn to Play* program

	Content	Underpinning skills
Foundation program	Attuning to your child	Attuning to the child is fundamental to the *Parent Learn to Play* program and is influenced by the child-centred play therapy approach of Axline (1947). Children are accepted for who they are and parents are taught to understand their child's play from the child's point of view.
	Sequencing play actions	The remaining content of the program is underpinned by the cognitive developmental theories of play. Each of the remaining skills is important in the development of the child's pretend play ability. Sequencing play actions logically occurs from approximately 24.

Table 9.1 Continued

Content	Underpinning skills
	months of age (Stagnitti, 1998). The ability to think logically is reflected in the pre-planning of sequential pretend play actions. Children begin to play in single acts (e.g. pretending to go to sleep), then in single acts with reference to another object (e.g. a doll), then they combine acts (e.g. the doll is put to bed and fed) (Stagnitti, 1998). By three years, children begin to pre-plan play acts in a sequence. By four and five years, children can sequence increasingly complex play actions with the addition of subplots (Westby, 1991). Children with ASD usually present with no pretend play sequences or limited action sequences
Describing the play	Talking about the play as you play has been referred to as 'metaplay' (Pellegrini and Galda, 1993). Metaplay and talking through conflicts during pretend play have been found to be important in understanding stories. Describing what the child is doing in the play not only gives the words for the play but conveys to the child that the parent is interested in what they are doing.
Object substitution	Object substitution is using an object and pretending it is something else. It is using symbols in play. Object substitution is a key feature of pretend play and is related to language.
Decentration	This is the ability to use an object outside of self – such as using the teddy as a separate being to the child. It is when a child imposes meaning and beliefs on an object that is separate to the child.
Play scripts	The stories in the play are play scripts. For children over 36 months, a short narrative is expected to be carried out in the play (Lewis *et al.* 1992). For four-year-olds, more complex

Table 9.1 Continued

Content	Underpinning skills
	social adjustments and sequences which incorporate sub-plots occur (e.g. telephoning the doctor because the baby was sick) (Westby, 1991). Play scripts are narratives and in this respect are parts of the child's literacy abilities. Play scripts also reflect the representation of themselves in their world.
Role play	Playing a character infers that you know how that character acts, what that character is likely to say, what motives the character has and what the character's beliefs are (Westby, 1991). Being able to role-play a character is a reflection of the child's understanding of their social and cultural world.
Intermediate program — Attributing properties	Attributing properties is when the child refers to the doll as 'sick', 'hungry', 'tired', 'angry', 'happy' and so on. This aspect of play usually involves imposing an emotional meaning on the play. It builds the context of the play scene.
Object substitution	See above. This skill is repeated as it is a core skill of being able to represent meaning in the play.
Reference to absent objects	By 3 ½ years, children have established the meaning of an object or action so well that they do not need the physical prop to play. Children can create a vision of what they are doing.
Adding problems to the play narrative	In understanding a narrative, a child understands character-appropriate language and behaviour such as a characters' actions, motives and goals that are consistent with a particular story (Westby, 1991). Children add problems to the play story because children play to a level that is challenging and interesting to them. It is part of the process of play and their engagement in

Table 9.1 Continued

Content	Underpinning skills
	the play. This part of the program is also about making the play more complex and challenging, and developing problem solving with resolutions.
Predicting what will happen next	When children understand narrative they can think forward, they can think into the future. This skill is also about understanding divergent problem solving, in that there can be many solutions and endings to a story. It is part of the unpredictability of play.

For the *Parent Learn to Play* program to be effective, the key principles are:

1. The child is accepted for who they are. While the adult begins by modelling a play skill, the adult responds to the child.
2. Start on the child's developmental play level. It is very important to begin where the child is. Measures of pretend play are the Symbolic and Imaginative Play Developmental Checklist (SIP-DC) (Stagnitti, 1998); Child-Initiated Pretend Play Assessment (ChIPPA) (Stagnitti, 2007); The Test of Pretend Play (Lewis and Boucher, 1997); and the Symbolic Play Scale (Westby, 1991). When working with children with autism or developmental difficulties I have found that it is not uncommon for these children to be two to four years delayed in their pretend play development. For example, a child of 5 years can be on the 18 months level for his pretend play. By starting on the child's play level, you are starting on a meaningful level to the child.
3. Use variation with repetition. When children enter the program and their play is developmentally below the 3 year level, it is important to use lots of repetition within the play activity and also for this repetition to vary. Repetition is very important because the more children engage with the play activity the more they begin to understand it. For example, within a tea-party scene you don't just have one cup of tea but many cups of tea, as long as the child is engaged; you keep having cups of tea but you vary it slightly each time. For example, you might have a sip, then you might offer a taste to teddy, then you might sip, then you might stir the cup and then sip, then you might blow on the tea because it is hot. Each time you are having a cup of tea but it is slightly different. Children with difficulty in their play need this repetition so that they can process what you are doing. You are building up the context of the play.

4. The focussed attention of the child is essential. By focussed attention I mean that the child is looking and is interested in what you are doing. They are focussed on what is being played out. For children with autism I do not expect them to look at my face but I do encourage them to look at my hands and look at the toys. If they are looking at my hands or the toys then they are seeing the play that is being carried out. I find as children with autism become involved in the play and in the process of play, they will look at me and engage in eye contact with me.
5. Talk about the play as you are playing. Pellegrini and Galda (1993) call this 'metaplay'. Talking about the play as you play gives the child the language for the play and builds up narrative language. I have interpreted Doidge's (2010) discussion of Hebb's theory and Merzenich's theory as giving a neurological explanation of why it is important to talk about the play as you carry it out. Essentially, according to Doidge, if two neurons are fired repeatedly at the same time they will connect more strongly and this can be influenced by experience. So, in play if you talk about the play as you are playing, then the play action and the language will connect more strongly. In play, you are also engaging with the child in social interaction, talking about the play and playing, so you are firing together language, social interaction, and play. I have found that after 7 sessions of the *Learn to Play* program, children show increased language and social turn taking and these are noticed by parents and adults outside the play sessions (Stagnitti and Casey, 2011).
6. You emotionally engage and genuinely enjoy playing with the child. Emotional engagement through play is more powerful than just going through the motions of play. When children become emotionally engaged in the play, they show greater understanding of the play in subsequent sessions (Stagnitti and Casey, 2012). The emotional engagement gives them greater understanding of the play. Sunderland (2007) discusses the importance of caring and loving a child and contrasts the brain scans of children who were in orphanages who were physically but not lovingly cared for with children who were lovingly and physically cared for. The brain scan of the child from the orphanage showed inactive areas in the temporal lobes, which 'can result in poor social and emotional intelligence' (p. 52), whereas the scan of the child who had received loving parenting showed fully active and dense connections in the temporal lobes. Engaging with children in a caring way during play embeds the play more meaningfully for the child.
7. The interaction with the child is permissive in that the child is free to initiate their own ideas. Self-initiation of play means the child understands their play and this is meaningful for the child.

Children who have been part of the *Parent Learn to Play* program all have a story to tell. Below are the stories of three of them.

Jack

Jack was diagnosed with autism when he was 3 years old. His parents had been considering a behavioural program but decided that the Parent Learn to Play *program would give their son valuable play skills. While his parents valued play they were not confident in how to engage Jack in play and Jack was difficult to engage. It was like he lived in a bubble; that is, he was in his own world and showed little enjoyment in engaging in play. He loved characters from movies and television and these characters were often used to attract Jack's attention within the play. After the seventh week, which was introducing object substitution within the play, I spoke with his dad about the session. Jack was distracted and didn't seem to be fully focussed for a lot of the session. His dad said that Jack was really interested in Lightning McQueen®, a story about a racing car. We decided that for the parent-run object substitution session we would create racing cars out of boxes. The boxes were large enough to step into and you could pull up the boxes to the waist. Jack was very engaged in the play and the play sequences allowed for lots of repetition with variation such as racing, crashing, sleeping, going in a truck to the next race, racing, sleeping and so on. Dad was one of the cars and his car helped Jack's car. Dad prompted the play, followed Jack's lead in the play, and put boundaries around when needed. Jack remained in his bubble state for several months and his ability to spontaneously sequence his play actions remained at four actions; however, other aspects of his play were changing. For example, he could refer to absent objects, he began to put problems in the play, he could use a teddy or character in the play and give them their own thoughts and he could attribute properties. Jack started to understand narrative and Dad began to joke with him in the sessions with Jack responding with a smile. In the last session, Jack laughed and chuckled with the puppets and created a magic show. He took over the play and acted with a freedom he hadn't shown for most of the year. Dad said that he was starting to show an interest in other children and was calling to them over the fence to come and play. He went to school the following year and understood the context of school and what was expected. By his second year of school he was part of a peer group.*

Robert

Robert showed no play ability on his initial play assessment. When I placed a truck on the floor he stepped over it and sat down to play with his screen toy. His mother was distressed that he needed entertainment all day and she felt guilty when she put on television for him to watch so she could make dinner. Robert had a diagnosis of intellectual disability and autism. On the first play session for sequences of play actions, the first activity was a toy dog feeding out of a bowl (1 action). As Robert's mum was a vet and Robert had a dog at home, starting with dog feeding was within Robert's experience. When I placed the dog's mouth to the bowl it was immediately clear that Robert was not interested. His mum took the dog and jumped it all over Robert in a similar manner to what his dog did at home. Robert giggled and laughed, at first responding to the feel of the dog and the tickling. After ten minutes of the dog jumping over him, Robert started to realise that it was the dog that was jumping on him. When this shift occurred, I asked mum for the dog and put its face in the bowl. Robert was very interested. He had focussed attention. After the dog had a long drink in the bowl it jumped on him again and then had another drink. This happened three more times and then the play activity was changed. After five sessions, his mum quietly explained that Robert had played on his own for one hour. He had never done this before. His mum was delighted and moved. By the end of the Parent Learn to Play session, Robert had moved from no play ability to being able to self-initiate his own play and continue in domestic play scripts with his sister for two hours most days of the week. His mum understood where his play ability was and could adjust her interaction and respond to his cues and extend his play without going to a level where Robert lost interest.

Billy

Billy screamed and screamed on his first session. His mum explained to me that he thought I was going to give him a needle. As he was experiencing me as a threat, I remained across the room from him while mum calmed him down. When I brought out a toy I gave it to mum and suggested how to use the toy to engage Billy's attention. By the end of the session he was giving his mum toys and gesturing that she play with him. As Billy was two years old, his play sequences were short and so play activities were repetitive with short action sequences. At first, mum tended to dominate the play but after modelling and gentle suggestions on alternate ways to engage Billy in play, mum could respond to Billy, accept his play ideas, and add to his play in a way that engaged him further. He can now re-direct his attention when he is given limits within the play room. He adores his mum and, during all sessions, he now deliberately engages his mum in play with her responding to him in his play ideas.

Conclusion

Play is often used as a measure of the level of attachment of a child to a parent. Children with ASD often present with disorganised attachment styles and have difficulties with pretend play. While their parents are sensitive to their needs, these children often respond to their parents in ways that do not reciprocate their parents' care. By developing a child's play and showing parents how to engage with their child in play, parents find a safe place in which to enjoy their child for who they are. Improvements in a child's play through the program are accompanied by improvements in language and social understanding. Future research into the *Parent Learn to Play* program will include work with parents who are struggling with their parenting, who have experienced generational poverty and who themselves have not played as children.

Key points

1. Parents with children with ASD show parental sensitivity.
2. Children with ASD come into the program with delayed pretend play skills which results in them presenting as disorganised in play.
3. Once children with ASD begin to self-initiate their play, they engage their parents in play.
4. The *Parent Learn to Play* program provides a safe place for parents to learn about the play of their child and how to engage with their child in play.
5. As children with ASD learn how to play, they show enjoyment and laughter in their interactions with their parents.

References

Ainsworth, M., Blehar, M., Waters, I. and Wall, S. (1978). *Pattern of Attachment*. Hillsdale, New Jersey: Erlbaum.
Axline, V. (1974). *Play therapy*. New York: Ballantine Books.
Bowlby, M. (1982 [1969]). *Attachment and Loss: Volume 1 – Attachment*. New York: Basic Books.
Doidge, N. (2010). *The Brain That Changes Itself*. Melbourne: Scribe.
German, T. P., Niehaus, J. L., Roarty, M. P., Giesbrecht, B. and Miller, M. B. (2004). Neural correlates of detecting pretense: automatic engagement of the intentional stance under covert conditions. *Journal of Cognitive Neuroscience*, 16 (10), 1805–17.

Green, J., Stanley, C., Smith, V. and Goldwyn, R. (2000). A new method of evaluating attachment representations in young school-age children: the Manchester Child Attachment Story Task. *Attachment and Human Development*, 2 (1), 48–70.
Lewis, V. and Boucher, J. (1997). *The Test of Pretend Play*. London: Psychological Services.
Nabor, F., Bakermans-Kraneneburg, M., van IJzendoorn, M., Swinkels, S., Buitelaar, J., Dietz, C., van Daalen, E. and van Engeland, H. (2008). Play behaviour and attachment in toddlers with autism. *Journal of Autism and Developmental Disorders*, 38, 857–866.
Norrie McCain, N., Mustard, F. and Shanker, D. (2007). *The Early Years Study 2: Putting science into action*. Ontario: Council for Early Child Development.
Pellegrini, A. and Galda, L. (1993). Ten years after: a reexamination of symbolic play and literacy research. *Reading Research Quarterly*, 28, 162–175.
Sherratt, D. and Peter, M. (2002). *Developing Play and Drama in Children with Autism Spectrum Disorders*. Oxon, UK: Dave Fulton Publishers.
Stagnitti, K. (1998). *Learn to Play: A program to develop the imaginative play skills of children*. Melbourne: Coordinates Publications.
Stagnitti, K. (2004). Understanding play: implications for play assessment. *Australian Occupational Therapy Journal*, 51, 3–12.
Stagnitti, K. (2007). *Child-Initiated Pretend Play Assessment*. Melbourne: Coordinates Publications.
Stagnitti, K. and Casey, S. (2011). Il programma *Learn to Play* con bambini con autismo: considerazioni pratiche e evidenze. *Autismo Oggi*, 20, 8–13.
Stagnitti, K. and Cooper, R. (eds) (2009). *Play as therapy: assessment and therapeutic interventions*. London: Jessica Kingsley Publishers.
Sunderland, M. (2007). *What Every Parent Needs to Know*. Dorling Kindersley: London.
van IJzendoorn, M., Rutgers, A., Bakermans-Kranenburg, Swinkels, S., van Daalen, E., Dietz, C., Naber, F., Buitelaar, J. and van Engeland (2007). Parental sensitivity and attachment in children with autism spectrum disorder: comparison with children with mental retardation, with language delays, and with typical development. *Child Development*, 78 (2), 597–608.
Vygotsky, L. S. (1966). Play and its role in the mental development of the child. *Voprosy psikhologii*, 12, 62–76.
Vygotsky, L. S. (1997). *Thought and Language*. (A. Kozulin, trans.) Massachusetts: The MIT Press.
Westby, C. (1991). A scale for assessing children's pretend play. In C. Schaefer, K. Gitlin and A. Sandrund (eds) *Play Diagnosis and Assessment*. New York: John Wiley and Sons Inc.
Wheatley, J. (2013). A different kind of miracle. *The Saturday Age Good Weekend*. Melbourne: Fairfax Media Publications. 18 May.
Whitehead, C., Marchant, J., Craik, D. and Frith, C. (2009). Neural correlates of observing pretend play in which one object is represented as another. *SCAN*, 4, 369–378.
Whitebread, D., Coltman, P., Jameson, H. and Lander, R. (2009). Play, cognition and self-regulation: what exactly are children learning when they learn though play? *Educational and Child Psychology*, 26, 40–52.

10

Group Theraplay®

Evangeline Munns

History and applications of family and group Theraplay

Theraplay was founded in 1967 by Dr. Ann Jernberg, a psychoanalytical psychologist from Chicago, Illinois, in response to a federal grant that she had received to increase the attachment between Head Start mothers and their children. These families often had single parents and lived in poverty. Just surviving was a challenge. Dr. Jernberg turned to the work of Dr. Austin DesLauriers (Booth and Jernberg, 2010) who had developed an unusual therapy working with schizophrenic children and those on the autism spectrum. His method was non-verbal, he ignored bizarre behaviour, concentrated on the children's strengths, was playful and action oriented and led the activities. Dr. Jernberg, a student of his (along with Dr. Viola Brody, founder of Developmental Play Therapy) incorporated his model and added an emphasis on physical contact and meeting the child at his/her emotional age. Today, Theraplay is practiced around the world. It is applicable to a wide age range (infants to the elderly) and to a variety of social, emotional and behavioural problems – i.e. dysregulated, aggressive, acting out, mute, withdrawn (Di Pasquale, 2009; Manery, 2000; Eyles *et al.*2009), but is especially helpful where there are relationship and/or attachment difficulties such as those found with adopted and foster children (Lindaman and Lender, 2009), step-children, failure-to-thrive infants (Bernt, 2000) and those on the autism spectrum (Goodyear-Brown, 2009). In addition, Theraplay has been used in marital therapy (Munns, 2009).

Group Theraplay was introduced by Phyllis Rubin, a speech pathologist and Janine Tregay, a teacher who wanted to create a sense of family in her special education class (Rubin and Tregay, 1989). Group Theraplay was at first adapted for peer groups ranging in age from preschoolers to the elderly involving various populations such as multi-cultural (Atkinson, 2009; Perry and Sunderland, 2009; Siu, 2009; Franke, 2009; Manery, 2000), children on the autism spectrum (Bundy-Myrow, 2000), children with physical and/ or intellectual disabilities (Azoulay, 2000), residential children (Buckwalter and Finlay, 2009) and juvenile delinquents (Gardner and Spickelmier, 2009). In addition, parent/child Theraplay groups evolved, such as a two family format including siblings (Sherman, 2000), multiple families with up to six parent/child dyads (Sherman, 2009), with adoptive parents and their children (Finnell, 2000), with Head Start mothers and their children (Zanetti *et al.* 2000), father/son groups (Sherman, 2009) and homeless mothers and their children (Rubin, 2000). Locations varied from school settings (Martin, 2000), to daycare and nursery school centres, to primary health care centres (Talen, 2000), to child mental health agencies, hospitals and shelters.

Additional characteristics

Theraplay is short term (the family or group is seen on a weekly basis for approximately 12 to 24 sessions, or more for complex clients), is cost effective (no toys or expensive materials or equipment needed), is non-verbal (no interpretations are made, but the child's feelings may be reflected), focuses on the positive strengths of the child and is physical, joyful and fun.

Theory

Theraplay is a model of play therapy based on attachment theory. Its main goals are to enhance the attachment between parent and child, to raise the self-esteem and confidence of both, to increase trust, to help the child self-regulate and to aid parents in becoming more attuned and responsive to their children's needs. Theraplay is based on replicating healthy normal parent/child interactions. The child is met at her/his emotional age, which in troubled children is often younger than their chronological age. Thus, at the beginning of treatment, activities are often geared to what a parent might do with a younger child. Theraplay goes back to the roots of connectedness and tries to fill in the gaps that might have been missed (Munns, 2009).

Underlying dimensions

In Theraplay, therapists focus on four underlying dimensions: *structure, engagement, nurture and challenge*. Certain dimensions are emphasized depending on the needs of the child – i.e. *structure* (which provides predictability, organization and safety) for children who are impulsive, acting out, defiant, uncooperative and/or dysregulated; *engagement* (which focuses on making connections and enjoyable interactions) for withdrawn, shy or depressed children; *nurture* (which emphasizes warmth, caring, soothing) for all children, but particularly for those who have been abused or neglected; and *challenge* (which focuses on mastery and confidence building) for those who have been overprotected, are timid and/or afraid to take risks. The therapist focuses on the child's strengths and ignores any bizarre behaviour. If the child does not want to do an activity then the therapist may use humour, paradox or diversion to gain cooperation, *but does not force the child.*

Research for family and group Theraplay

Theraplay is evidence based, but needs more studies using randomized control groups (Wardrop and Meyer, 2009). Those using randomized control groups or matched controls have shown that Theraplay helps to reduce aggression (Wettig *et al.* 2006; Franke, 2007; Lender and Lindaman, 2007), raises self-esteem and lowers internalizing symptoms (Sui, 2009). Other studies using control groups (non-randomized) have indicated increases in social emotional functioning and language expression (Ritterfeld, 1989) and increases in empathy of young, single mothers (Ammen, 2000). There are many more studies using pre versus post scores (but lacking control groups) showing an increase in attachment scores between parents and their children (Wardrop and Meyer, 2009), lowering of autistic symptoms (Franklin, 2007; Cross and Howard, 2007), lowering of the stress hormone (cortisol) (Lassenius-Panula and Makela, 2007) and lowering of aggression and externalizing behaviour (Munns *et al.* 1997). There are a considerable number of other research studies that are still in progress and/or have not been published (personal communication with the Theraplay® Institution). Clearly, more Theraplay studies using randomized control groups are needed, including groups utilizing other therapeutic interventions, are needed in order to control for the placebo effect. (This is a criticism from the author's viewpoint that can be applied to the whole field of play therapy.)

Supportive research

Brain research

Theraplay is supported not only by its attachment underpinnings, but also by some of the latest brain research. The activities incorporated into Theraplay sessions help to stimulate the right hemisphere of the brain, which is the first hemisphere to mature and is dominant until three years of age. The right hemisphere is non-verbal, creative, processes social emotional experiences and is sensory based (Cozolino, 2010). The right hemisphere is also important in affect regulation which is a key factor in the development of attachment (Schore, 2005; Schore and Schore, 2008) and self-regulation (Munns, 2011b). Theraplay activities help to stimulate and organize the lower brain which controls our survival systems including heart rate, breathing, digestion, body temperature and sexual urges. Our instinct to fight, flee or freeze in the face of danger is part of the lower brain and is triggered by connections to the amygdala in the emotional brain (limbic system). The amygdala is the 'watch dog' of the emotional brain and judges whether or not the environment is threatening or dangerous. It is overactive in children who have been chronically abused, often leaving them in a hypervigilant state with higher core temperatures and breathing rates. In Theraplay many activities are geared to calm and soothe these children as well as helping them to feel valued, important and cared for (Munns, 2011a).

Many Theraplay activities involve movement and rhythm which are controlled by the cerebellum of the lower brain. The cerebellum has strong connections to the amygdala and has dopamine receptors which can give a sense of pleasure and joy when stimulated by movement or rhythmic experiences. This helps to explain why music and rhythm can bring such an emotional response to many individuals. This also helps us understand why rhythm (rocking) is successfully used all over the world to soothe and calm young children.

Dr. Bruce Perry's neurosequential program (Perry and Szalavitz, 2006; Szalavitz and Perry, 2010) which has been used successfully with severely traumatized clients is congruent with the Theraplay approach. In the first part of his therapeutic program for clients with early trauma histories, when stimulating the lower brain Dr. Perry uses massage, dancing, movement, drumming and Theraplay activities.

Touch research

One of the main characteristics of Theraplay is its emphasis on positive, physical touch. This is based in part on Dr. Jernberg's observations of normal parents with their young children where there was a lot of physical contact (Booth and Jernberg, 2010). The parents interacted with their young children through holding, caressing and patting them, rocking, bathing, and nursing them, playing games such as 'patty cake', etc. Research with animals and humans has indicated the importance of touch for the well-being and normal development of children (Field, 2000; Gerhardt, 2004; Nicolson and Parker,

2009; Sunderland, 2006). The tactile sensory system is the most advanced sensory system in the newborn. If the infant does not receive touch it will not thrive (Nicolson and Parker, 2009). Both animal studies and research with human infants have shown this. Dr. Tiffany Field (2000) has done extensive, well-controlled research using massage. In one of her studies she randomly assigned premature human infants to a treatment group that received massage for 15 minutes, three times a day. The treatment group and the control group both received exactly the same amount and type of food. After ten days the massaged group significantly increased in body weight by 47 per cent, and left the hospital six days earlier than the control group. Dr Field has conducted numerous studies with various groups, including juvenile delinquents who showed significantly less aggression after receiving massage and ADHD children who were able to concentrate and focus better after receiving massage. In 1983, in South America, Dr Martinez and Dr. Rey had parents of premature babies carry their babies so there was skin to skin touch; results showed a 41 per cent drop in mortality rates within the treatment group and the parents felt closer to their babies as compared to the control group. Since then, there have been many research studies verifying the positive results for both babies and parents of this skin to skin method now referred to as 'kangaroo care' or 'baby wear' (Feldman *et al.* 2002; Ruiz-Pelaez *et al.* 2004). Other researchers like Thayer (1998) in correlational studies, have reported that countries that have the least amount of positive, physical touch amongst family members are associated with the highest rates of violence. Nicolson and Parker (2009) have suggested that if children are deprived of positive touch, they may turn to using aggressive touch (pushing, shoving and pinching).

North Americans tend to live in a 'touch phobic' world where people are generally afraid to touch others for fear of being accused of sexual misconduct or harassment. Therapists are advised not to touch their clients. Teachers are forbidden to touch their students, even young children when they are upset. In the past, students could not touch each other in an aggressive way, but now some schools in both the US and Canada are not allowing children to positively touch each other – i.e. no hugging. With the daily influence of watching violence depicted on TV and in video games, might our children be learning that aggression is more acceptable in our culture than physical affection? This is a question that needs to be addressed more fully in our society.

Group Theraplay

Various formats have been used with Theraplay: individual child, individual child and parents, whole families including all siblings, multiple families, peer groups and parent/child groups. This chapter focuses on the latter two groups.

Goals

Common to all groups are goals to raise the self-esteem and confidence of the participants, to increase social skills such as sharing and taking turns, to create a sense of cohesion and belonging, a sense of connection with others, to increase emotional expression appropriately and to experience laughter, fun and joy.

Group format

Groups have included up to eight children if they have behavioural, social or emotional problems (larger groups of up to 30 children have been included in normal school, kindergarten or daycare settings). It is wise not to have a majority of children (if possible) who are behaviour disordered, because the group can get too chaotic. It is also imperative to have a co-leader, especially when there are many impulsive, acting out children. The ages of the children should be fairly similar, ideally within a two year range.

The length of time of each group session varies according to the age of the children. Preschoolers may find it difficult to engage for more than 20 minutes while older children can be fully involved for 45 minutes to an hour. The total number of sessions varies – usually approximately 12 sessions at which point the goals and progress are re-evaluated. The group may continue or end depending on the progress of its members.

An agenda is pre-planned according to the needs of the children. Approximately nine to twelve activities are included and led by the leaders, but vary according to each age group and the length of each activity. A balance of active versus calm activities are incorporated. Certain dimensions are emphasized according to the needs of the group – i.e. more structured activities for a group of impulsive, externalizing children or more challenging ones for an adolescent group.

Certain activities are always included in all groups, such as: a welcome song or handshake, a quick inventory or checkup of participants' positive physical features at the beginning of the group, a powdering or lotioning of 'hurts' on the hands and a feeding of a favorite snack. Three rules are stated near the beginning by the leader in the first few sessions: 1 – 'no hurts', 2 – 'stick together' 3 – 'have fun'. However, the activities pertaining to each of the dimensions (structure, engagement. nurture and challenge) are changed each week.

Discipline

Disciplinary problems are handled in a sensitive, but firm manner. If the leaders notice that a child has been hurt intentionally or accidentally, the leader immediately stops the group, reminds the group that no hurts are allowed, and tries to find out what happened. The victim is asked to show where he/she has been hurt. The leader then states something like this: 'we have to look after that hurt. Let's see if we can make it better' – maybe giving a soft rub around the hurt, or putting on a band aid. The leader initiates the action, but also asks the aggressor to help rub the hurt gently. This helps the aggressor to make some kind of meaningful restitution. He/she is not asked to apologize, because that is often pointless. However, in helping to repair the hurt, the aggressor feels he/she has been part of the caring and not just caused the problem. The victim is encouraged to tell the aggressor: 'Don't hurt me anymore'. Meanwhile the aggressor is asked for his side of the story – was he troubled by anything? Whatever the reason, the leader tries to understand the motive of the aggressor. The act of restitution is powerful and may be one of the factors as to why, in research studies, Theraplay seems to reduce the amount of aggression (Wettig *et al.* 2006; Munns *et al.*, 1997). Anecdotal reports from teachers and therapists are numerous and cite many instances where former 'bullies' are now one of the first to try to care for the child that has been hurt (personal communication from Arruda (2013), who at present is leading 17 Theraplay groups in schools in northern Alberta, Canada). The first kind of group that will be described will be a peer group followed by a parent/child group.

Peer group

Makeup of group
The group consisted of eight children, nine to ten years of age with a range of emotional and social difficulties (from withdrawn and mute, to acting out and disobedient). Some were learning disabled but were within the normal range of intelligence. Two were extremely bright and easily got restless and bored.

This group met once a week in the afternoon for approximately 30 minutes in a classroom. At the beginning parents had met in a group to discuss the goals of the group. Theraplay was described and written parental consents for treatment and videoing were obtained. Plans for having 12 sessions were discussed, with a re-evaluation at the end. Evaluation questionnaires such as the Achenbach Child Behaviour Scale were filled out by the parents and teachers pre and post groups.

Agenda

A typical agenda for the above group (activities varied from session to session) was:

Entrance: Follow the leader (children line up at the door, behind the leader who makes a series of maneuvers that the children imitate – i.e. big steps, little steps, slow, fast, etc. ending in a big circle facing inwards).

Welcome (hello song or handshake): Everyone holds hands while the welcome song that includes each child's name is sung: 'Hello Johnny, hello Sally, hello Jimmy we're glad you came to play', etc.

Check up or inventory: The leader kneels in front of each child and notices one special positive feature re each child ('Hi Karen, I see you've brought your bright, blue eyes today', 'Steve, you've brought your wonderful smile', 'David, I can see that dimple in your chin', etc.). This is done quickly as the leader moves around the circle.

Three rules: 'Remember our three rules: no hurts, stick together and have fun!'

Powdering or lotioning of hurts: Leaders put baby powder or lotion on the cuts, bruises, red spots, (boo-boos) on the hands of each child. (Leader and co-leader attend about 4 children each.) In later sessions the children sometimes lotion the 'hurts' of each other.

Dimensions: Four or more activities from the dimensions of structure, engagement, challenge and nurture are then played out, for example:

- 'Red light, green light' (structure). Children move forward in a line when the leader says 'green light' and stop when the leader says 'red light'. If a child is caught moving during 'red light' then he/she must move back to the starting line.
- 'Balloon toss' (engagement). Leader calls a child's name and then tosses a balloon to them. That person then tosses the balloon to someone else while calling out their name. This continues until every name has been called. Then several balloons are tossed in the air that everyone tries to keep up in the air.
- 'Pass a gentle touch' (nurture). Leader begins by gently touching the shoulder of his/her neighbour and this contact is passed around. Each child then initiates a gentle touch that is passed around.
- 'Duck, duck, goose' (challenge). All are sitting except for 'it', the person that walks around the outside of the circle while touching each

child's head saying 'duck'. When the 'it' person instead says 'goose' the child he has just touched immediately gets up and runs in the opposite direction. When the 'goose' and 'it' meet, they either shake hands or give each other a quick hug and then continue running until they get to the spot 'goose' has just vacated. Whoever gets to that spot last, is the next 'it'.

- 'Bean bag hug' (nurture). All children are sitting as a bean bag is passed around while the group chants: 'one potato, two potato, three potato four, five potato, six potato, seven potato more'. Whoever gets the bean bag on the word 'more' is then given a hug by his/her neighbour on either side. The game continues until each child is hugged.
- 'Feeding of a snack' (nurture): Leaders feed each child potato chips, pieces of fruit, etc. Several rounds of food are given around the circle. In later sessions children sometimes feed each other.

Good-bye song: Everyone sings a simple song that includes each child's name – i.e. 'Goodbye David, goodbye Tim, goodbye Leslie, we're glad you came today. Goodbye Kim, goodbye Sally, goodbye Johnny, we're glad you came today', etc. until each member's name is mentioned (or, sometimes with adolescents, a special goodbye handshake).

Ending statement: We'll see you all next week at the same time and the same place, Wednesdays at 3pm.

Evaluation

This group continued for 12 sessions and a post evaluation by teachers and parents indicated that there was less acting out, less impulsivity, less aggression and more sensitivity to others including an awareness of when a child was hurt. There were more frequent comments such as 'Get the baby powder out – Sally has been hurt'. Teachers also felt the children started to know each other's names sooner. Some of the children who had been 'bullies' were not being aggressive anymore and at times would even be caring to other children. The teachers also felt that they had become closer to the children.

Parent/child group

Parent/child groups have ranged from mother/child, father/child to multiple family groups (Munns, 2009). One of the plans (that has not yet materialized for the present author) of having a group that involved grandmothers, their daughters and grandchildren, will some day in the future, hopefully, address the transmission of intergenerational patterns of attachment more directly.

The following is a description of a father/son group:

Makeup of group

The group consisted of six father/son dyads with two male leaders. The boys ranged in age from five to thirteen years (not an ideal range). This group included several children with their step-fathers, two children with Asperger's syndrome, and several acting out, aggressive children including a 13-year-old who was in a treatment residence for severely troubled clients. The latter had expressed his anger by punching holes in the walls of his room. All of the fathers were married, employed and came from a middle class socio-economic level. The group met once a week for two hours; one hour for Theraplay followed by one hour of parent counselling and debriefing. During the parent counselling, the children were taken by the co-leader to play games outside if the weather was suitable, or inside for handicrafts, storytelling or games. Before the group started, all of the fathers met with the leaders to discuss the nature of Theraplay and its goals. The fathers contributed their ideas for group goals and two goals emerged that were common to all of the fathers:

- I want my son to be more obedient and cooperative.
- I want to be closer to my son.

A typical agenda for this group follows.

Agenda

Entrance: everyone lines up behind the leader who pretends he is an airplane bending from side to side as he strides into the room with everyone following him. They end in a circle facing inwards.

Getting acquainted: 'Name Whip' – every person takes a turn calling out his name while turning his head to the right.

Welcome song: Leader starts singing a song mentioning each person's name: 'Hello Johnny, hello Mac, hello Sam, we're glad you came to play', etc.

Three rules: Leader quickly talks about the three rules: 1. 'no hurts' (physical or verbal) 2. 'stick together' (do whatever the leader is asking them to do) 3. 'have fun'.

Inventory: The boys first form a circle sitting outward while each father kneels in front of his son. Each father notices three or four special, positive features of his son – e.g. strong shoulders, nice ears, brown, sparkling eyes, shiny dark hair.

Caring of hurts: The fathers lotion or powder the hurts of their child's hands.

Making shapes: Each child turns his back to his father who traces a shape (circle, square, triangle, etc.) on his child's back with his finger using a firm touch. After the child guesses the shape, the father rubs out the shape by sweeping his hand back and forth across his child's back before tracing another shape. At the end, the father gives his child a back rub.

Motor boat: Everyone gets up and walks in a circle to the right while singing: 'Motor boat, motor boat go so slow, motor boat, motor boat go so fast, motor boat, motor boat run out of gas'. At this point everyone sits down.

Peanut butter-jelly: The leader calls out 'peanut butter' and the group answers back 'jelly' in exactly the same pitch, tone and pace of the leader who varies how he calls out 'peanut butter' each time (e.g. fast, slow, soft, loud).

Cotton ball guess, fight, soothe: Children kneel in a straight row facing their fathers who are also kneeling in a straight row about two feet apart from their sons and then do the following activities:

> *Cotton ball guess*: Each father touches his son with a cotton ball on various parts of his body (face, hands, shoulders etc.) while the child, with his eyes closed, guesses where he has been touched.
>
> *Cotton ball fight*: Rows spread further apart (about three or four feet). A bunch of cotton balls is placed in front of each person. When the leader calls out 'go' everyone throws a ball at anyone, but calls out that person's name first. When the leader calls out 'let her rip' everyone can throw as many balls as they want at anyone without calling his name first. (This often creates a lot of fun and laughter.)
>
> *Cotton ball soothe*: Rows come closer together so fathers can reach out to their sons to soothe their faces by gently, but firmly, rubbing their forehead, nose, chin, jaw etc. with a cotton ball while their son receives this touch with eyes closed. Fathers can comment positively while they are doing this – strong jaw, straight nose, nice ears, etc.

Feeding: While in a circle, each father is given five or six potato chips (or pieces of fruit, etc.) that he feeds to his child. Sometimes, the leaders feed everyone (including the fathers) several rounds of chips.

Goodbye song: Everyone holds hands and sings the name of each individual – 'Goodbye Henry, goodbye Jeff, goodbye Hal, we're glad you came today, etc.' (to a simple tune).

As mentioned before, the fathers remain for debriefing and counselling while their children go out to play. The children are given juice and cookies before they leave, while the fathers are served coffee and cookies. (Serving food is part of nurturing and is often as important to the fathers as it is to the children.)

Evaluation

In the group described above, there was almost 100 per cent attendance for the 12 sessions, even when there was bad weather in the winter. Children would insist on coming even if they were ill. Some fathers commented that this group was the most special time in the week for them, where there were no other distractions to spending time with their sons. One of the positive outcomes of this group was the spontaneous affection observed between the fathers and sons. There was an obvious increase in 'feeling closer'. Additional benefits were the growing friendships forged within the group. Previously all of the children had social skill difficulties and a lack of friends. Within this group, children started to spontaneously invite each other to their birthday parties and overnights. One father and son lived on a farm and invited the whole group for a day's adventures on their farm one weekend.

The leaders felt that, if allowed, this group could have gone on indefinitely. Generally, everyone was reluctant to finish. However, due to a long waiting list, and the fact that many of the referral problems of the children had improved, only two families were included in the next group.

Conclusion

Group Theraplay can be used effectively for all ages – from infants, toddlers, latency-aged, adolescents, adults and the elderly – and for a wide variety of emotional, social and behavioural difficulties. These include the externalizing, aggressive children, as well as the shy, mute, withdrawn, depressed children and those on the autism spectrum. It is cost effective and short term (often only 12 sessions are needed). It can be used in a variety of formats – peer, parent/child, family and couple groups. The goals are to enhance the self-esteem and confidence of all the participants, to increase their trust and enjoyment of each other, to increase the social skills of sharing and taking turns and, most importantly, to feel connected with others and to have a sense of belonging. In parent/child groups, the most important goal is to enhance the attachment between parent and child so that they can feel delight and joy in being with each other.

Key points

1. Theraplay is an attachment enhancing form of play therapy.
2. It is short term and cost effective.

3. It replicates normal parent/child interactions.
4. It can be used for all ages and for a wide range of emotional, social and behavioural difficulties.
5. Group Theraplay can be used in a variety of formats: peers, parent/child, families, and couples.
6. It is evidenced based, but needs more randomized control groups in research studies.

Note

Theraplay is a registered service mark of The Theraplay® Institute, Evanston, IL, USA.

References

Ammen, S. (2000). A play-based parenting program to facilitate parent/child attachment. In H. Kuduson and C. Schaefer (eds) *Short term play therapy approaches for children* (pp. 345–369). New York: Guilford Press.

Arruda, M. (2013). Personal communication. Northern Alberta, Canada

Atkinson, N. (2009). Theraplay used in a multi-cultural environment. In E. Munns (ed.) *Applications of family and group Theraplay* (pp. 137–157). Lanham, MD: Aronson.

Azoulay, D. (2000). Theraplay with physically handicapped and developmentally delayed children. In E. Munns (ed.) *Theraplay: Innovations in attachment-enhancing play therapy* (pp. 279–300). New York: Aronson.

Bernt, C. (2000). Theraplay with failure-to-thrive infants and mothers. In E. Munns (ed.) *Theraplay: Innovations in attachment-enhancing play therapy* (pp. 117–137). Northvale, NJ: Jason Aronson.

Booth, P. and Jernberg, A. (2010). *Theraplay: Helping parents and children build better relationships through attachment-based play.* San Francisco, CA: Jossey-Bass.

Buckwalter, K. and Finlay, A. (2009). Theraplay: The powerful catalyst in residential treatment. In E. Munns (ed.) *Applications of family and group Theraplay* (pp. 81–93). Lanham, MD: Aronson.

Bundy-Myrow, S. (2000). Group theraplay with children with autism and pervasive development disorder. In E. Munns (ed.) *Theraplay: Innovations in attachment-enhancing play therapy* (pp. 301–320). New York: Aronson.

Cozolino, L. (2010). *The neuroscience of psychotherapy: Healing the social brain.* New York, NY: W. W. Norton and Co., Inc.

Cross, D. and Howard, A. (2007). *An evaluation of Theraplay with children diagnosed with PDD or mild to moderate autism.* Paper presented at the third International Theraplay Conference, Chicago, IL.

Di Pasquale, L. (2009). The dysregulated child in Theraplay. In E. Munns (ed.) *Applications of family and group Theraplay* (pp. 27–44). Lanham, MD: Aronson.

Eyles, S., Boada, M. and Munns, C. (2009). Theraplay with overtly and passively resistant children. In E Munns (ed.) *Applications of family and group theraplay* (pp. 45–55). Lanham, MD: Jason Aronson.

Feldman, R., Weller, A., Eidelman, A. and Sirota, L. (2002). Comparison of skin-to-skin (kangaroo) and traditional care. Parenting outcomes and preterm infant development. *Pediatrics*, 110, 1, 16–26.

Field, T. (2000). *Touch*. Cambridge, MA: MIT Press.

Finnell, N. (2000). Theraplay innovations with adoptive families. In E. Munns (ed.) *Theraplay: Innovations in attachment-enhancing play therapy* (pp. 235–256). New York: Aronson.

Franke, U. (2007). *An analysis of the therapeutic treatment process using Theraplay with oppositional, defiant children and shy, withdrawn children.* Paper presented at the third International Theraplay Conference, Chicago, IL.

Franke, U. (2009). Theraplay in Germany. In E. Munns (ed.) *Applications of family and group Theraplay* (pp. 127–136). Lanham, MD: Aronson.

Franklin, J. (2007). *An evaluation of Theraplay using a sample of children diagnosed with pervasive developmental disorder (PDD) or mild to moderate autism.* Paper presented at the 21st National Conference on Undergraduate Research, San Raphael, CA.

Gardner, B. and Spickelmier, M. (2009). Working with adolescents. In E. Munns (ed.) *Applications of family and group Theraplay* (pp. 249–264). Lanham, MD: Aronson.

Gerhardt, S. (2004). *Why love matters: how affection shapes a baby's brain.* New York: Brunner-Routledge.

Goodyear-Brown, P. (2009). Theraplay approaches with children with autism spectrum disorders. In E. Munns (ed.) *Applications of family and group Theraplay* (pp. 69–80). Lanham, MD: Aronson.

Lassenius-Panula, L. and Makela, J. (2007). Effectiveness of Theraplay with Symptomatic Children Ages 2–6: Changes in Symptoms, Parent-child Relationships, and Stress Hormone Levels. Paper presented at the Third International Theraplay Conference, Chicago, IL.

Lender, D. and Lindaman, S. (2007) *Research supporting the effectiveness of Theraplay and the Marschak Interaction Method.* Paper presented at the third International Theraplay Conference, Chicago, Illinois.

Lindaman, S. and Lender, D. (2009). Theraplay with adopted children. In E. Munns (ed.) *Applications of family and group Theraplay* (pp. 57–68). Lanham, MD: Aronson.

Manery, G. (2000). Dual family theraplay with withdrawn children in a cross-cultural context. In E. Munns (ed.) *Theraplay: Innovations in attachment-enhancing play therapy* (pp. 151–194). New York: Aronson.

Martin, D. (2000). Teacher-led theraplay in early childhood classrooms. In E. Munns (ed.) *Theraplay: Innovations in attachment-enhancing play therapy* (pp. 321–337). New York: Aronson.

Munns, E. (2009). *Applications of family and group Theraplay*. Lanham, MD: Aronson.

Munns, E. (2011a). Theraplay: Attachment enhancing play therapy. In C. E. Schaefer (ed.) *Foundations of play therapy* (2nd edn) (pp. 275–296). Hoboken, NJ: Wiley.
Munns, E. (2011b). Integration of child centered play therapy and Theraplay. In A. Drewes, S. Bratton and C. Schaefer (eds) *Integrative play therapy* (pp. 325–340). Hoboken, NJ: Wiley.
Munns, E., Jensen, D. and Berger, L. (1997). *Theraplay and the reduction of aggression.* Unpublished research, Blue Hills Child and Family Center, Aurora, Ontario.
Nicholson, B. and Parker, L. (2009). *Attached at the heart.* New York: iUniverse.
Perry, B. and Szalavitz, M. (2006). *The boy who was raised as a dog.* New York: Basic Books.
Perry, L. and Sunderland, P. (2009). Theraplay and aboriginal peoples. In E. Munns (ed.) *Applications of family and group Theraplay* (pp. 97–114). Lanham, MD: Aronson.
Ritterfield, U. (1989). Theraplay auf dem prufstand. Bewertung des therapieerfolgs am beispiel sprachauffalliger vorschulkender (Putting Theraplay to the test: evaluation of therapeutic outcome with language delayed preschool children). *Theraplay Journal,* 2, 22-25.
Rubin, P. (2000). Multi-family Theraplay groups with homeless mothers and children. In E. Munns (ed.) *Theraplay: Innovations in attachment-enhancing play therapy* (pp. 211–234). New York: Aronson.
Rubin, P. and Tregay, J. (1989). *Play with them – Theraplay groups in the classroom: A technique for professionals who work with children.* Springfield, IL: Thomas.
Ruiz-Pelaez, J., Charpak, N. and Cuervo, L. (2004). Kangaroo-mother care: An example to follow from developing countries. *British Medical Journal,* 329 (7475), 1179–1181.
Schore, A. (2005). Attachment, affect and the developing right brain: Linking developmental neuroscience to pediatrics. *Pediatric Review,* 26, 204–217.
Schore, J. and Schore, A. (2008). Modern attachment theory: The central role of affect regulation in development and treatment. *Clinical Social Work Journal,* 36, 9–20.
Sherman, J. (2000). Multiple family Theraplay. In E. Munns (ed.) *Theraplay: Innovations in attachment-enhancing play therapy* (pp. 195–210). New York: Aronson.
Sherman, J. (2009). Father-son group Theraplay. In E. Munns (ed.) *Applications of family and group Theraplay* (pp. 237–248). Lanham, MD: Aronson.
Siegel, D. and Hartzell, M. (2003). *Parenting from the inside out.* New York, NY: Jeremy P.Tarcher/Putman.
Siu, A. (2009). Theraplay in the Chinese world: An intervention program for Hong Kong children with internalizing problems. *International Journal of Play Therapy,* 18, 1, 1–12.
Sunderland, M. (2006). *The science of parenting.* New York: DK Publishing.
Szalavitz, M. and Perry, B. (2010). *Born for love.* New York: HarperCollins Publishers.

Talen, M. (2000). Using Theraplay in primary health care centers. In E. Munns (ed.) *Theraplay: Innovations in attachment-enhancing play therapy* (pp. 339–361). New York: Aronson.

Thayer, T. (1998). March Encounters. *Psychology Today*, 31–36.

Wardrop, J. and Meyer, L. (2009). Research in Theraplay effectiveness. In E. Munns (ed.) *Applications of family and group Theraplay* (pp. 17–24). Lanham, MD: Aronson.

Wettig, H., Franke, U. and Fjordbak, B. (2006). Evaluating the effectiveness of Theraplay. In C. Schaefer and H. Kaduson (eds) *Contemporary play therapy* (pp. 103–135). New York: Guilford Press.

Zanetti, J., Matthews, C. and Hollingsworth, R. (2000). Adults and children together (ACT): A prevention model. In E. Munns (ed.) *Theraplay: Innovations in attachment-enhancing play therapy* (pp. 257–275). New York: Aronson.

11 How neuroscience can inform play therapy practice with parents and carers

Theresa Fraser

> Understanding how the brain develops, what fosters or hinders this development, the potential impact of both, and how to use this information to provide corrective developmentally appropriate experiences is at the heart of a neurosequential approach to play therapy.
> (Prendiville, 2013)

Introduction

When working with children who have experienced developmental trauma, it is vital that we take a systemic approach, giving due consideration to findings from contemporary research surrounding neuroscience. In this chapter I will explore ways to appropriately engage children and their carers in family play therapy sessions where an understanding of relevant neuroscience underpins my work. I will begin by giving a brief overview of brain development and the factors that influence this. I will then look at planning and delivering interventions guided by neuroscientific evidence, and provide a case study vignette.

Development of the brain

The development of a child's brain can be impacted upon by many factors and the first vulnerable stage of development is whilst the child is *in utero*. Exposure to alcohol or drugs *in utero* can have lifelong consequences;

for example, in the case of fetal alcohol syndrome, also known as alcohol related neurobehavioural disorder (Streissguth and Kanter, 1997)

The physiological and psychological effects associated with domestic violence or other external stressors have also been linked to the health of the newborn's brain. Horner (2005) states that infants can be born prematurely, and/or have lower birth weight, as a direct result of their mother's emotional stress and/or experiences of physical trauma. In addition, perinatal care directly impacts the development of the brain stem which can cause sensory integration problems, hyper-reactivity, poor state regulation (e.g. sleep, feeding, self-soothing) and tactile defensiveness as well as problems with the regulation of core neurophysiological functions such as breathing and temperature regulation (Perry, 2009, p. 9).

The brain is divided into four major parts which develop and become more organized and complex over time. First the brainstem (hindbrain), then the diencephalon (midbrain), followed by the limbic system and, finally, the cortex (forebrain). The brainstem, comprised of the midbrain, pons and medulla, regulates bodily functions. The midbrain manages vision, hearing, involuntary movements and body movements. The pons acts as a motor relay centre by receiving and sending messages to and from the cerebrum (thought action) and cerebellum (motor control). Swallowing, facial expressions, bladder control, facial sensations and sleep are regulated by the pons. The medulla manages circulation, breathing and heart rate. Midbrain connections create templates in response to regular experiences that drive our reactions to, or reasoning about, incoming experiences. As learned responses, these templates can become an operating mode for the child when they are presented with similar sensory experiences in the future.

The diencephalon and the limbic system are responsible for our emotional functioning. The diencephalon comprises the thalamus and the hypothalamus, both essential for the regulation of behaviour and emotion (Mash & Wolf, 2010). The hypothalamus regulates biological needs such as thirst and hunger. The limbic system helps to organize the child's emotions. It builds on midbrain functions in relation to attachment, affiliation with others, motor regulation, emotional reactivity and sexual behaviour (Perry, 2009). The limbic system is connected with all the major body systems.

Lastly, the cortex manages the most complicated tasks, including decision-making, interpersonal communication, empathy, attention span and impulse control. This part of the brain 'allows us to look to the future, and plan, to reason and to create' (Mash and Wolfe, 2010, p. 41).

All parts of the brain function in orchestration with each other. Communication within the brain occurs via neurotransmitters and synapses. Synapses are junctions where neurons pass signals to other neurons using neurotransmitters. Perry and Szalavitz (2006) describe neurotransmitters as keys that open synaptic locks. 'All experiences are recorded, encoded and recalled through synapses. It is through sets of synapses that individual thoughts become linked as concepts or tied to specific events' (Rothschild, 2000, p. 19).

In the face of neglect or trauma, areas of the brain that are already organized (e.g. lower parts such as the brainstem) are not as responsive to environmental stimulation and repetition; they are no longer as malleable as higher levels of the brain, such as the cortex. The already organized and functional neural system is less vulnerable to trauma than a system that is still in development (Perry, 2009).

Factors that can foster or inhibit brain development

What happens in the world outside of the child at key developmental periods impacts on the development of the brain. During early childhood, the organizing neural networks require touch, sight, sound, smell and movement in order to develop normally (Perry, 2013). Maturation of the brain is experience dependent. In order to support the growth of children, we need to create responsive, nurturing and enriching life spaces. Time spent ensuring this is of most importance early in life (Perry, 2013). The mother's mental health status directly impacts her baby. Infants and toddlers absorb information via their senses and learn about relationships and social interactions through their life experiences. These experiences influence their emotional stability and worldview. For example, if they are living in domestic violence situations they may expect all social interactions to be violent or aggressive (Baker and Cunningham, 2004) and, as such, this template provokes their stored response of alarm (Perry, 2001).

A healthy environment for children requires the absence of stress evoking experiences and the enhancement of co-regulating experiences to support healthy attachment between baby and caregiver. Much has been written about the life-long effects of babies being neglected and ignored. As is argued by Szalavitz and Perry (2010), the quality of the interaction between a baby and their primary care giver is the most fundamental predictor of healthy brain development. 'Just as physical punishment hurts a child's feelings, as well as her body, so emotional neglect damages the whole child even though she is outwardly well cared for' (Leach, 2010: 485).

The stress hormones adrenaline, noradrenaline and cortisol, also impact the growing child. When the child experiences fear or terror, the amygdala recognizes threat and sends a message to the hypothalamus. The hypothalamus releases a hormone (corticotropin) that communicates to the pituitary gland to release another hormone (adrenocorticotropic). This triggers the adrenal gland to produce cortisol which, in sustained and elevated levels, can become toxic to the brain (De Bellis, 2005; Rees, 2010; Siegel 2012). In the absence of nurturing and soothing, the child functions in a stress based, self-preservation mode which can manifest itself in physical, psychological and behavioural difficulties (Courtois, Ford and Briere, 2012).

Considering trauma

The National Institute for Trauma and Loss (Steele and Raider, 2001; 2009) categorizes trauma into three types:

1. a single event, such as a car accident or sexual assault
2. a repeated event, such as being sexually abused by the same perpetrator
3. also known as complex trauma, this is categorized as many traumatic experiences as well as various kinds of traumatic experiences.

Children who have experienced varied, long term and invasive traumatic experiences are impacted on many levels, including their ability to attach and connect relationally with others. Their emotional thoughts and responses may not match the expectations of others, their behaviour might appear to be out of sync with events that are precipitatory, they may dissociate (freeze) and their self-concept and future orientation can be impaired.

Children who have experienced complex trauma, including exposure to domestic violence, neglect, emotional abuse, physical abuse and/or sexual abuse, present differently in different circumstances and with different people. They might present as being ultra-mature at times, yet regress emotionally on occasion, in ways associated with a much younger child. They may have no awareness of how their behaviour impacts on family members, pets or friends, perhaps appearing to purposefully hurt others when, in reality, doing what they believe they need to do to survive. Their template response to anxiety-provoking events might be a fight, flight or freeze response (Levine, 1997). For example, newly placed children who have lived in domestic violence environments may not be able to answer questions asked of them or may answer 'no' to all questions regardless of the content (Fraser, 2011). They may be hyper-alert to visual environmental cues because they are suspicious of adult caregivers and are highly skilled at assessing environmental threats in order to survive. 'Dysfunctional symptoms and functional assets in children are both related to the nature, timing, pattern and duration of their developmental experiences' (Perry and Hambrick, 2008, p. 40).

Many children who present for therapy, particularly children who are within the care system, have trauma histories that fall into the complex trauma category. Adults may observe a myriad of unusual behaviours and responses to even minor stressors. There is a neurological basis for these learned responses – just as attuned caregiving has a positive impact, trauma negatively impacts on brain, personality development and attachment.

> The child's constitution, temperament, strengths, sensitivities, developmental phase, attachments, insight, abilities; the reactions of his loved ones; and the support and resources available to him, all contribute to how an event is experienced, what it means to the child, and whether or not it is traumatizing at that specific time in the child's life.
> (James, 1989, p. 2)

Using the neurosequential model of therapeutics to plan interventions and intake sessions

Once trauma has occurred, individual intervention can include a combination of play therapy, psycho-educational intervention, cognitive behavioural approaches (that might also be trauma focused), insight orientated therapy and pharmacotherapy. Given that 'trauma refers to overwhelming, uncontrollable experiences that psychologically impact victims by creating in them feelings of *helplessness, vulnerability, loss of safety*, and *loss of control*' (James, 1989), interventions need to focus on assisting the child to feel strong, to feel safe and also to feel empowered. Trauma informed interventions could result in containing the acting-out behaviour that often undermines the stability of the placement for the child in care. Play can assist the child in expressing non-verbally their view of the world as well as their view of the relationship shared with caregivers. This will assist the child in moving from feeling vulnerable to knowing that he or she will be cared for. Both child-centred and focused play therapy approaches can assist a child in being able to negotiate with others in appropriate ways for the purpose of meeting their needs. Feelings of helplessness can be replaced with those of competence. Another treatment goal that can be met by family play therapy is to assist the child to have increased positive encounters and attachment experiences so that they can move from feelings of loss of safety to knowing that they can be a cared for child in a healthy parent/child relationship.

The Neurosequential Model of Therapeutics (NMT) is not a specific intervention but, rather, an approach to clinical work that is informed by neuroscience (Perry, 2008). The model places priority on assessing the child's development and resources in relation to their history and life experience in order to establish whether, where and/or to what extent, disrupted or distorted brain development may have occurred.

Play therapists understand the importance of working from a developmental and multi-systemic perspective with individuals, including children, who have experienced trauma. This includes understanding the impact of their history and gathering information about their current functioning, and any current challenges within their systemic world (Brendtro, 2006). Bidirectional influences can support or undermine therapeutic interventions so informed clinicians will use a trauma informed approach to engage with carers when treating child clients. An understanding of relevant neuroscientific findings, specifically an understanding of how the brain develops and is affected by abuse, neglect and trauma, can be invaluable in our work. Enhanced practice using NMT can ensure that developmentally appropriate corrective interventions can be applied.

At the intake stage of service it is helpful for the play therapist to meet with parents or primary clinicians so the therapist can ascertain how things are going for the child in his/her many life spaces. It is good practice for clinicians to spend time gathering information to inform the treatment roadmap, especially with children who have had multiple primary caregivers. Often there is much that is unknown about the child's early history, including both challenges and protective/resiliency factors. All adults who work with the child can benefit greatly from using a trauma focused lens to look beyond the presenting behaviours, connecting 'symptoms' with the child's traumatic exposure, and/or neglectful, experiences. Using NMT we are able to link a child's presenting behaviour with the area of the brain that was actively developing at the time of the traumatic experience.

> [T]he *specific* dysfunction will depend upon the timing of the insult (e.g. was the insult *in utero* during the development of the brainstem or at age two during the active development of the cortex), the nature of the insult (e.g. is there a lack of sensory stimulation from neglect or an abnormal persisting activation of the stress response from trauma?), the pattern of the insult (i.e. is this a discreet single event, a chronic experience with a chaotic pattern or an episodic event with a regular pattern?)
>
> (Perry, 2001, p. 9)

Sharing resources with the parent can be especially helpful as they often lack awareness of the impact of the child's early trauma history, particularly if the child has lived with them for a significant amount of time. Adoptive parents commonly believe that the child should feel safe because the child's safety, physical or emotional needs are now addressed and they are not currently being abused.

To heal the hurt child, one begins not as a clinician but as a person trying to witness how the child experiences trauma. This requires more than just talking since the child's terrifying experiences are stored in the brain's senses and visual imagery, not in rational thoughts and words. The goal is to change these frightening sensory experiences which hold the child hostage.

(Steele, 2008, p. 44)

The fact that children are impacted in both the short and long term as a result of trauma and attachment disruption experiences is a beginning point of reference when working with new primary caregivers of children who have experienced developmental trauma (whether they are adoptive, foster, kin parents or group home staff).

The home environment

In relation to Perry's work with the children of a cult in Waco, Texas, Perry and Szalavitz (2006) reported that children needed to have times during their day to process their experiences at their own pace and in their own ways. The opportunity to talk with an adult was available if a child wanted or, in the safe space of play, they could develop new childhood memories, offsetting their earlier, fearful ones (p. 71). Fraser (2011) proposes a four stage model to guide the creation of a healing environment for the child which comprises: Structure; Safety; Supervision; and Support.

Safety

Children need to have consistent physical, emotional, and sexual safety rules. These should be in place when a child is newly placed in a care environment so that the rules and routines do not appear to be born of mistrust of the child who has a sexual or aggressive acting-out history. It is easier to decrease expectations after a child is settled in a milieu than to increase expectations later.

Structure

Structure speaks to creating predictability in the child's life and ensuring that all adults who interact with the child are using similar language, responses and are essentially consistent with expectations. Home routines need to be predictable but parents may also have to advocate that appointments occur on the same day of the week or time of day. These children often do not manage transitions well, hence parents (with the help of their play therapist) may need to advocate for school meetings so staff are made aware of the importance of their role in helping the child feel safe at school. Fewer rotary classes and changes in learning environments may help the child be more successful in the school milieu.

Supervision

Supervision for children who have been neglected may initially feel constrictive given they may not be accustomed to family focused activities and meals. Repetition will ease this discomfort so supervision does not feel punitive. Parent/child relationships improve when children begin to have developmentally appropriate supervision. There is time for play and interaction throughout the day.

Support

Lastly, the support in the four S's is for the primary caregivers or helpers. We all need supportive networks – helpers of children who have been traumatized, especially, need to have supports in place. These should take the form of time with their partner, time working on hobbies and time with other adults who care and parent kids with complex trauma histories. The play therapist should be mindful of the need for peer support groups and make appropriate referrals for these or facilitate these so parents are gaining their own much needed support. Being able to normalize your personal or familial experiences helps caregivers to be creative. Front-end planning and environmental preparation decreases the use of consequences that at times feel like they do little but to acknowledge to others in the milieu that a specific behaviour was unacceptable.

Promoting the development of self-regulation

Relaxation exercises, or stress management, need to be introduced to child and family so this process can be repetitively practiced and supported outside of the therapy room. Vickhoff *et al.* (2013) found that the heartbeats of singers in a choir become synchronized, hence singing in the company and in rhythm of others is good for your health! This is no surprise to clinicians who utilize Theraplay® as an intervention to help child and parent interact in synchronicity. Once a child is able to calm physiologically, they can then find the words to express how they are feeling. Often, however, the child with a complex trauma history lacks emotional literacy and may need some therapy time focused on connecting words to feelings and feelings to experienced physical states. Later (often much later in the therapeutic process), they can begin to connect triggers to their experienced physical states. This is especially true for children who have experienced pre-verbal trauma. They do not have the words to explain why they feel the need to run and hide or scream, fight or dissociate from the here and now. Language is tied to explicit memory. The healing work must focus on helping the child to connect self-care strategies that can be implemented when their body is sending a specific message. The cause of the physiological response can be a future consideration.

Often children have struggled with appropriate expression, so this is an important part of the process. Helping parents understand the importance of creating a supportive environment is paramount here, rather than focusing on behaviour management strategies. Children require a safe, predictable environment and will respond more successfully to this as compared to sticker charts and concrete reinforcers for pro-social behaviours (James, 2013).

The play therapy environment

The PRACTICE acronym summarizes the Trauma Focused Cognitive Behavioural Therapy (TF CBT) process:

- Psycho-education and parenting skills
- Relaxation
- Affective expression and regulation
- Cognitive coping
- Trauma narrative development and processing
- *In vivo* gradual exposure
- Conjoint parent-child sessions
- Enhancing safety and future development.

(Gateway, 2012)

Cognitive coping can help to lay foundation for the creation of a trauma narrative. This is an essential part of the process, assisting the child in recognizing the impact of the trauma experience on them but that also their role was that of a victim. Cognitive reprocessing is the next stage. If there are sensory triggers associated with the trauma, the therapist may need to create *in vivo* opportunities for mastery and, where possible, include the primary caregiver in understanding the process that the child has experienced. Lastly, future planning with the child and caregiver needs to occur so the child recognizes that they are now residing in a different and safer world. This will take repetitive reassurance that their needs will be met. TF CBT can involve play therapy interventions during each stage of the process. This will include direct teaching and bibliography in addition to strategies and techniques such as game play, drumming, music, dance or progressive muscle relaxation (which can be utilized to model and teach relaxation as well as affective expression and regulation). In a 2012 study, 158 children aged 4–11 years were treated using the TF CBT approach and their improvements continued even after 6–12 months of treatment completion (Mannarino *et al.* 2012, pp. 231–241). The trauma focused play therapist has to be aware that the later stages of PRACTICE require cortical brain functioning.

Using NMT to guide direct work with the traumatized child

Perry (2009) identifies that patterned neural activation is necessary for neural re-organization. This can include music, movement and yoga (for breathing) and drumming or therapeutic massage for state-regulation. Parents can utilize infant massage techniques to help the child become more in touch with their body, breathing, heart rate, etc. The play therapist can incorporate somato-sensory integration activities into sessions, encouraging the child's awareness and control over rhythm. This can improve links between higher and lower brain regions (Perry and Szalazitz, 2006). Once this is achieved, then the child may be ready to proceed to relational problems (limbic) using more traditional play and art therapies. Once dyadic relationship skills are established, therapeutic techniques can become more insight orientated (cortical) using a variety of Cognitive Behavioural or psychodynamic approaches (Perry and Hambrick, 2008, p. 42).

Neuroscience suggests that play, if not play therapy, is essential to the recovery of children who have experienced trauma and attachment disruptions (Perry, 2001). Many models of play therapy focus on facilitating repetitive experiences. Perry talks about assisting the child to develop new 'templates' about their world and those in it (Perry, 2006, p. 33).

Neural systems respond to prolonged and repetitive activation by altering their neurochemical and micro architectural (e.g. synaptic sculpting) organization and functioning (Perry, 2001: 20). Therefore, if the child experienced trauma and/or neglect in infancy when the brainstem was organizing, they may benefit from play experiences that are repetitive such as drumming and rocking. (Many North American therapy rooms have rocking chairs available for clients to utilize in the healing space.) Outside of the therapy room, the child may be a great candidate for massage therapy or parent/child touch activities can be integrated into a formal Theraplay protocol or directive activities that help to establish state-regulation are scheduled at the beginning of the play therapy session.

If the child requires midbrain stimulation, the therapist can be mindful of sensory integration and enrichment activities such as music making or aromatherapy. Movement activities such as dance, yoga and gymnastics – even if these are provided outside of the play therapy space – will provide enrichment. In order to address or enhance limbic system functioning, play activities can help to facilitate and enhance emotional regulation. Activities to facilitate this might include dance, play with natural materials, creative arts and play therapy.

Case study

Martin was a three-year-old who was being adopted by his paternal grandfather and his wife of ten years. They had provided ongoing support to the birth mother who had lived all of her life with her mother while only visiting her father on alternate weekends or for extended periods when conflict with her mother became dramatic. As a teenager, Martin's mother, although depressed, experimented with drugs and alcohol and was sexually promiscuous. She hid her pregnancy from her parents for many months and was suspected of continuing to self-medicate using alcohol and drugs while pregnant. She had ongoing arguments with her mother, both before and after Martin was born, that at times precipitated police intervention. She had a boyfriend living with her and her mother. All three, and the boyfriend's parents, would often engage in verbal conflicts, particularly when family members were drinking. Martin's mother verbalized that he was a difficult baby and would drop him off at her father's home regularly and then disappear for days at a time. He was apprehended at two years of age by the local child protection agency and ultimately placed with his paternal grandfather and his wife for the purpose of adoption.

He slept little, tantrumed often, and was described by his adoptive parents as needing to control everything at home (e.g. television viewing, seating arrangements). He was aggressive with the family cat, slow in his speech development and uncomfortable with physical closeness, such as cuddling. This therapist first met Martin and his parents in their home and was able to make suggestions about environmental routines prior to the family participating in a Marschak (MIM) assessment (Jernberg and Booth, 2010). He was also referred to a developmental paediatrician in order to gain insight into his developmental functioning and presentation. Theraplay occurred for ten sessions, focusing on structure and nurture with adoptive mum and child.

Activities included drumming, singing, blanket swings and stack of hands. The next phase of treatment included a registered massage therapist being brought in to teach adoptive mum how to utilize infant massage for a little boy who clearly was impacted by his environment both in utero and as an infant when his brain was attempting to wire at the state regulation stage. We then continued to incorporate somato-sensory integration activities both in and outside the play therapy room using music, art-based and physical activities such as utilizing a small trampoline. Adoptive mum registered him in a jungle gym programme as well as a toddler's music program that she co-participated in initially. Later she was able to observe from the parent observation areas.

For home enrichment, this therapist recommended activities such as blowing bubbles and making Kool-Aid play dough and other activities so that Martin was experiencing repetitive sensory experiences. In the play therapy room he would spend non-directive time in the sand, usually choosing big trucks while making truck sounds. His choice of world toys was not surprising given that his adoptive dad was a long distance truck driver.

Emotional regulation activities were focused on to support limbic brainwork, both in the therapy room and at home, utilizing a filial approach with special playtime between mother and child. At four years of age his adopted mother provided psychoeducation to staff of a new nursery program so that they were aware of Martin's need for routine, predictability, support during transition times as well as music and movement programming. Overall his treatment included providing him and his mother with a variety of approaches including directive, non-directive and prescriptive (Gil, 2006; Goodyear-Brown, 2010), and tools in order to assist him to get to the point where mother could help him to self-regulate. His sleeping improved, his relational connection with his parents improved, tantrums decreased and speech improved. Both parents successfully utilized Theraplay activities at different stages of their daily routines and this helped Martin be in control of himself as well as to feel safe with his parents (Jernberg and Booth, 2010).

Bath (2008) proposes that trauma informed care should focus on three pillars: safety, connections and managing emotions. Adults who are supporting children with complex trauma experiences can create environments that address these areas outside of the play therapy room in order to support the work of the play therapist in the play therapy room. Martin's adoptive mother was able to create safety as well as provide her son with supportive

Table 11.1 A neurodevelopmental approach to case conceptualization and treatment planning

Hypothetical case details	Presenting issues	Potential impact on brain development	Neurodevelopmentally appropriate intervention
Whilst pregnant, Lauren was physically and emotionally assaulted by her partner Paul. The abuse continued through to the birth although Lauren did not report it for several months, by which time her baby, David, was 4 months old.	Lauren generally has a low mood and minimal energy. She finds looking after David tiring. David is fed on demand and is always bathed and in clean clothing (in fact Lauren changes him many times a day). He does not sleep well, however, and is lower than average weight. He is fed on demand but his appetite seems low. He cries often and loudly and Lauren verbalizes difficulty in holding him given his anticipated fearful or angry cries whether he is being held or left to cry in his crib.	Trauma here may have impacted on the development of David's brain through the pregnancy due to the stress Lauren was under. In addition, at this early age, brain-stem development and the development of the diencephalon may have been impacted. These areas being associated with sleep and appetite.	Lauren is meeting David's basic needs but both Lauren and David would benefit from engagement in Theraplay®, that promotes touch and interaction – peek-a-boo, nursery rhymes or singing games can encourage this. David may also benefit from sensory stimulation and baby massage. In the absence of Theraplay®, a parenting skills programme/psychoeducation focusing on the importance of touch and attunement would be beneficial.
Ben was taken into care when he was 3 years old because of his mother's active alcoholism. She lost her partner, Ben's father, soon after Ben's first birthday and	Ben has started nursery school and the staff at the children's centre have noticed that he spends much of his time observing what is going on rather than taking part in activities. He appears 'clumsy', his solitary play is exploratory – picking	Trauma here may have impacted on the development of Ben's brain at a number of levels, particularly the midbrain, and delayed development of the	It might be useful for staff at the children's centre to be briefed about potential explanations for Ben's difficulties. In particular, discussion might focus on how trauma and the development of play are closely related and that

Table 11.1 Continued

Hypothetical case details	Presenting issues	Potential impact on brain development	Neurodevelopmentally appropriate intervention
although she had not drunk for 4 years she relapsed within 2 months of the funeral. Ben's needs were no longer consistently met when his mum started drinking. For example, he was once left alone for 16 hours until neighbours became alerted by his crying and secured entry to care for him. At this point the authorities became involved.	up toys, putting them into his mouth, shaking and banging them, and looking closely at them. He is easily distressed, rarely speaks to the staff or other children and avoids eye contact. While his mum says he was a good sleeper as an infant, this is no longer true. He often rocks in his crib to self-soothe. During meal times he will eat until he is sick so caregivers need to ensure that he is provided with appropriate portions. He eats quickly and is always looking around to compare what he has with the meals of other children. He will refuse help from staff or his foster parents. He will run out of the centre if upset but does not run to anywhere in particular. Music can be effective in soothing him.	limbic area. He appears to be presenting with difficulties associated with the limbic area demonstrating issues with social interaction and attachment. His under-developed play skills may be indicative of trauma associated with the midbrain.	mastering early forms of play is needed before more complex play can evolve. Routine and the repetition of activities will facilitate a sense of trust and predictability. Within the centre, the sensory play that Ben frequently engages in can be expanded (playing with both dry and wet substances and a variety of textures) and encouraged, adding opportunities for social interaction within this play. Adults can bring an air of playfulness to shared activities. Gross motor play should also be facilitated. Development of the midbrain might be encouraged through music and movement with a particular emphasis on rhythm and repetitive movements such as drumming or dance activities. Restricting the number of staff that he is negotiating and navigating relationships with will help him to begin to feel safe.

Antonia is an 11-year-old girl who is the second of four siblings. Though Antonia has lived in a loving adoptive home for four years she previously lived in two other foster homes after being taken into care at the age of five. Antonia's biological parents argued all the time. Mother had a substance abuse problem and moved to another part of the country away from her husband but with her four children to begin a new life. Antonia was often required to diaper and care for her younger twin siblings. Her older brother

Antonia's presenting problems appear to be a direct result of her early exposure to multiple complex trauma events as well as lack of exposure to age appropriate activities.

Antonia's adoptive parents sought therapeutic intervention because Antonia appeared very disorganized, left messes everywhere, avoided family mealtimes, would not accept help from her parents, and was very impulsive and easily angered. She wouldn't sleep in her own bed and was often observed to be self-harming after achieving low marks at school or being corrected at home. She had limited peer social skills and would isolate herself for long periods of time.

Given that Antonia's play skills and emotional functioning do not match with her chronological age and that her complex history is likely to have led to impairment in all areas of brain development, a comprehensive treatment plan is needed. This will include regular home-based interventions plus therapist-directed and facilitated play sessions, including self-directed play. Parental and therapist warmth and attunement to Antonia's emotional states will be important as will simple tracking and reflective commentary.

Antonia often functions emotionally at a level below that expected of an 11-year-old. Ascertaining and responding in a stage (rather than age) appropriate manner to her developmental functioning moment-to-moment will be important.

Antonia needs assistance to get in touch with bodily sensations. A stethoscope will be shared with the family with a plan for Antonia to first chart her resting heartbeat and then later her heartbeat when she is becoming agitated so as to help her recognize when she needs parental assistance and calming activities.

Hand or foot massages with baby lotion will help Antonia experience safe, nurturing touch.

Table 11.1 Continued

Hypothetical case details	Presenting issues	Potential impact on brain development	Neurodevelopmentally appropriate intervention
often watched pornographic television and all children observed their mother having relations with various men.	Antonia has not developed a connection with her adoptive parents as yet, although she has been placed with them for four years. They report that she often attempts to play them off against each other in order to be the person in the house who is in control. She approaches the parent who took parenting leave more readily. Antonia has broken many items around the home in anger, including items that are special to her.

Antonia had difficulty maintaining focus and attention. Projects and assignments were often unfinished or not handed in to her teacher when they were complete. Her teacher described her as being hyperactive and hypervigilant. | Interventions are intended to initially address the brainstem and midbrain area by focussing first on establishing state regulation through positive touch and repetitive sensory input. Music, rhythm and movement-based activities will increase somato-sensory integration. Antonia's needs in these areas are indicated by her lack of regulation, hypervigilance and persistent anxiety.

Later interventions will address limbic system deficiencies to improve emotional | Routines and repetition of activities in her school and home life spaces will provide consistency and predictability for Antonia.

Relaxation exercises and playing relaxing music may help Antonia to self-soothe at bedtime.

Antonia will benefit from a combination of Theraplay and non-directive play therapy sessions. Her adoptive parents can be part of these sessions at key times.

When the interventions at home, school and in play therapy sessions, show evidence in assisting brainstem and midbrain functioning, Antonia may be ready for limbic and cortical oriented approaches that |

She was reported to struggle with transitions both at school and home. She would become aggressive when she had to wait to get attention or to have a need met.	regulation and tolerance through art, play, and social activities.

Finally, story-based and dramatic activities will support cortical development and improve and increase Antonia's capacity for abstract thinking and insight. (Perry, 2006) | include art-based, drama-based and narrative work as well as bibliotherapy. This will include activities that focus on turn-taking and sharing. Expressive and creative materials such as art supplies, dress up clothes, puppets and sand tray will be provided, as will games with rules.

The therapist could present a trauma training workshop so that school staff can understand that Antonia's behaviour is often a coping style based on trauma history. |

J. Howard, E. Prendiville and T. Fraser, 2013

connecting relationships, all of which laid foundations for the child to be able to begin to regulate his emotions in various life spaces.

> In order to heal a damaged or altered brain, interventions must target those portions of the brain that have been altered. Because brain functioning is altered by repeated experiences that strengthen and sensitize neuronal pathways, interventions cannot be limited to weekly therapy appointments. Interventions must address the totality of the child's life, providing frequent, consistent replacement experiences so that the child's brain can begin to incorporate a new environment – one that is safe, predictable and nurturing.
>
> (Children's Bureau/ACYF, 2009, p. 13)

Key points

1. Trauma experiences and attachment disruptions interfere with neurobiological development.
2. Understanding the sequence involved in brain development is central in taking a developmentally appropriate approach to play therapy.
3. A systemic approach is necessary to achieve the best results for the child.

References

A lower brain connection. (2006). *Brain Highways*. Available online at www.brainhighways.com (accessed 1 May 2013).
Applegate, J. and Shapiro, J. (2005). *Neurobiology for clinical social work*. New York: W. W. Norton.
Axline, V. (1974). *Play therapy*. New York: Random House Publishing Group.
Baker, L. and Cunningham, A. (2004). *Supporting woman abuse survivors as mothers*. London, Ontario: Centre for Children & Families in the Justice System, London Family Court Clinic, Inc.
Bath, H. (2008). The three pillars of trauma informed care. *Reclaiming children and youth*, 17 (3), 17–21.
Brendtro, L. K. (2013). The vision of Urie Bronfenbrenner: adults who are crazy about kids. *Reclaiming children and youth*, 15 (3), 162–166.
Children's Bureau/ACYF. (2009). Understanding the effects of maltreatment on brain development. Available online at www.childwelfare.gov/pubs/issue_briefs/brain_development/brain_development.pdf (accessed 29 May 2013).

Courtois, C., Ford, J. D. and Briere, J. (2012) *The treatment of complex trauma: a sequenced relationship based approach*. New York: Guilford Press.

De Bellis, M. (2005). The psychobiology of neglect. *Child Maltreatment*, 10 (2), 150–172.

Franey, K., Geffner, R. and Falconer, R. (2001). *The cost of child maltreatment*. San Diego, CA: Family Violence and Sexual Assault Institute.

Fraser, T. (2012). *Adopting a child with a trauma & attachment disruption history*. Ann Arbor, MI: Loving Healing Press.

Gateway, C. (2012). Trauma-focused cognitive behavioral therapy for children affected by sexual abuse or trauma. Available online at www.childwelfare.gov/pubs/trauma/trauma.pdf (accessed 02 May 2013).

Gil, E. (2006). *Helping abused and traumatized children*. New York: Guilford Press.

Goodyear-Brown, P. (2010). *Play therapy with traumatized children*. Hoboken, NJ: John Wiley & Sons.

Horner, G. (2005). Domestic violence in children: effects of domestic violence in children. *Journal of pediatric health care*, 19 (4), 206–212.

Hughes, D. (2007). *Attachment-focused family therapy*. New York: Norton and Company.

James, A. (2013). *Welcoming a new brother or sister through adoption*. London: Jessica Kingsley Publishers.

James, B. (1989). *Treating traumatized children*. Lexington, MA: Lexington Books.

Jernberg, A. and Booth, P. (2010). *Theraplay: helping parents and children build better relationships through attachment based play*. San Francisco, California: John Wiley.

Leach, P. (2010). *Your baby and child*. London: Dorling Kindersley Ltd.

Levine, P. (1997). *Waking the tiger*. Berkeley, CA: North Atlantic Books

Malchiodi, C. (2008). *Creative interventions with traumatized children*. New York: Guilford Press.

Mannarino, A., Cohen, J., Deblinger, E., Runyon, M. and Steer, R. (2012). Trauma-focused cognitive-behavioral therapy for children: sustained impact of treatment 6 and 12 months later. *Child Maltreatment*, 17 (3), 231–241.

Mash, E. and Wolfe, D. (2010). *Abnormal child psychology* (4th edn). Belmont, CA: Wadsworth/Thomson Learning.

Munns, E. (2000). *Theraplay*. Northvale, NJ: J. Aronson.

Perry, B. D. (2001). The neuroarcheology of childhood maltreatment: the neurodevelopmental costs of adverse childhood events. In K. Franey, R. Geffner, and R. Falconer (eds), *The cost of maltreatment: Who pays? We all do* (pp. 15–37). San Diego, CA: Family Violence and Sexual Assault Institute.

Perry, B. D. (2006). The neurosequential model of therapeutics: applying principles of neuroscience to clinical work with traumatized and maltreated children. In N. B. Webb (ed.), *Working with traumatized youth in child welfare* (pp. 27–52). New York: Guilford Press.

Perry, B. D. (2009). Examining child maltreatment through a neurodevelopmental lens: clinical applications of the neurosequential model of therapeutics. *Journal of Loss and Trauma*, 14 (4), 240–255.

Perry, B. D. (2013). *Brief: Reflections on Childhood, Trauma and Society*. Houston, TX: Child Trauma Academy Press.
Perry, B. and Hambrick, E. (2008). The neurosequential model of therapeutics. *Reclaiming children and youth*, 17 (3), 38–43.
Perry, B. and Szalavitz, M. (2006). *The boy who was raised as a dog*. New York: Basic Books.
Prendiville, E. Approach Neurosequential to Play Therapy. Email message, 12 September 2013.
Rees, C. (2010). Understanding emotional abuse. *Archives of Disease in Childhood*, 95 (1), 59–67.
Rothschild, B. (2000). *The body remembers*. New York: Norton.
Schaefer, C. and Drewes, A. (2013). *The Therapeutic Powers of Play*. Hoboken: Wiley.
Schore, A. (2013). *Joy and fun, gene, neurobiology and child brain development*. Available online at www.youtube.com/watch?v=Y0iocZu1m (accessed 22 September 2013).
Siegel, D. (2012). *The developing mind: how relationships and the brain interact to shape who we are* (2nd edn). New York: Guildford Press.
Steele, W. (2008). Clinician or witness: the intervener's relationship with traumatized children. *Reclaiming children and youth*, 17 (3), 44–47.
Steele, W. and Raider, M. (2001). *Structured sensory intervention for traumatized children, adolescents, and parents*. Lewiston: Edwin Mellen Press.
Steele, W. and Raider, M. (2009). *Structured sensory intervention for traumatized children, adolescents, and parents*. Lewiston: Edwin Mellen Press.
Streissguth, A. and Kanter, J. (1997). *The challenge of fetal alcohol syndrome*. Seattle: University of Washington Press.
Swain, J., Lorberbaum, J., Kose, S. and Strathearn, L. (2007). Brain basis of early parent infant interactions: psychology, physiology and 'in vivo' functional neuroimaging studies. *Journal of Child Psychology and Psychiatry*, 48 (3–4), pp. 262–287. Available online at http://meteor.aihw.gov.au/contents index.phtml/itemId/327314 (accessed 26 May 2013).
Szalavitz, M. and Perry, B. (2010). *Born for love*. New York: William Morrow.
Vickhoff, B., Malmgren, H., Åström, R., Nyberg, G. F., Ekström, S., Engwall, M., Snygg, J., Nilsson, M. and Jörnsten, R. (2013). Music structure determines heart rate variability of singers. *Frontiers in Psychology*, 4.

Index

Page numbers in **bold** indicate tables and in *italic* indicate figures.

absorption in play 115–16
abuse: physical 66, 83, 182; puppets 104; sexual 66, 83, 182; *see also* domestic violence; neglect
Achenbach Child Behaviour Scale 170
acting-out behaviour 183
activities: distraction 55–8; domestic violence interventions 69–70; Group Theraplay 170–1, 172–3; NDP/EPR groupwork 91–4; outdoor play 119–26; post-procedural play 58–9; special dreams 55, 56, 57; *see also* puppets; stories
adjustment issues, and touchstone stories 13–15
affective dysregulation, and puppets 106–7
affect regulation 137, 166
aggression: and puppets 99–100, 109; and Theraplay 165, 169, 171; and touch 167
Ainsworth, M. 150
alcohol related neurobehavioural disorder 179–80
amygdala 39, 166, 181
anxiety 40, 83; and hospitals 47–8, 52, 55, 61; and puppets 99–100; and touchstone stories 9, 11
ASD *see* autism spectrum disorder (ASD)
attachment 114, 150–1; and the brain 166, 180, 181; and NDP/EPR 82, 83, 84; and Theraplay 164, 165

attachment difficulties 73, 163
attention 35, 40, 115, 121, 158
attributing properties 152, **156**
autism spectrum disorder (ASD) 133, 138; and attachment 150–1; pretend play 154; and puppets 101; and Theraplay 163, 165; *see also* Parent Learn to Play program
autobiographical self 35
autonomy 2–3, 49, 61, 71, 72, 73
Axline, V. 151–2, 153

baby wear 167
Barbie picnics activity 58–9
Bath, H. 195
beating the bounds activity 120–1
behavioural dysregulation, and puppets 106–7
behavioural effects of domestic violence 66, **67**
behavioural issues, and touchstone stories 10–13
body awareness *see* embodiment development
body-self 82–3
books, as distraction 55
bounded rationality 30–1
brain: amygdala 39, 166, 181; and consciousness 40; development 179–83, 190–4; lateral prefrontal cortex 40; learned feedback loops 39–40; memory 16, 18–19, 21, 40,

116, 123; mirror neuron system 139; and neglect 65, 181, 184, 188–9; and parent-child relationship 149–50; and pretend play 152–3; and Theraplay 165–6; and trauma 18–19, 181, 182–3
brainstem 180, 188
Braverman, L. D. 35
Broadhead, P. 2
Broca's area 18
bubbles, as distraction 55
Bush Tucker trials activity 59

case studies: consciousness 37–45; domestic violence 72–4; hospital play 51–4, 59–60; multiple disabilities 134–5, 136–7, 138; *Parent Learn to Play* program 158–60; puppets 52–4, 54, 99–101, 105–6, 107; trauma informed interventions 189–95
Cattanach, A. 75
cerebellum 166, 180
cerebral palsy 59, 134
characters, miniature 10, 22–3, 40–4
Chesner, Anna 135
child-centred play therapy 32, 151–2, 153, 183; *see also* non-directive play therapy
Child-Initiated Pretend Play Assessment (ChIPPA) 157
child protection procedures 65
cognitive coping 187
cognitive developmental theories of play 152, **154**
cognitive distortions 17–18, 104, 105
cognitive effects of domestic violence 66, **67**
cognitive reprocessing 187–8
compensatory play 72
competence, and puppets 100
complex histories: and touchstone stories 17, 20–1; trauma 182–3, 187, 195
confidentiality 12, 20
congruence 7, 24
consciousness 29–45; case study 37–45; models of 29–30, 34–7; Play Therapy Dimensions Model 30–4, *31*, 38
controlled breathing 58
control of play, child's 2–3, 49, 61, 71, 72, 73
core consciousness 35
core self 35
cortex 40, 180

cortisol 150, 165, 181–2
Cozolino, L. 114
creative groupwork: NDP/EPR 88–94; and puppets 104, 108–9; *see also* group sessions

Damasio, A. 35
dance 140–1, 189
Davis, D. 69
Davis, N. 108
decentration 154, **156**
decision-making 30–1; *see also* Play Therapy Dimensions Model
DesLauriers, Austin 163
development: brain 179–83, **190–4**; and domestic violence 66, **67**; embodiment 82–4, 113–16; and neglect 65; play 51, 132–3, 152, 153–4, **154–7**; relationship 91, 140–1; sensory 113–14, 122
developmental difficulties *see Parent Learn to Play* program
developmental play, in hospitals 49–52
diencephalon 180
directiveness dimension 31–2, *31*, 33
disabilities: effects on play 59; *see also* autism spectrum disorder (ASD); multiple disabilities
discipline, group sessions 90, 108–9, 168–9
disorganised attachment 150, 151
disruptive behaviours, and puppets 109
distraction techniques 55–8
dogs, fear of 39
Doidge, N. 158
dolls 52, 98, 151; attributing properties 152, **156**; miniature characters 10, 22–3, 40–4; worry dolls 69–70
domestic violence 64–75; effects of 66, **67**, 180, 181, 182; prevalence 64, 65; psycheducation 104; therapeutic play 68–74; and touchstone stories 16
dopamine 150, 166
dramatic distance: doll characters 9, 10, 22; puppets 98, 102, 110; stories 107
dramatic play 86–7; *see also* role play
dreams, special 55, 56, 57
dynamic psychiatry systems 34

educational play, in hospitals 49–52
electronic devices, as distraction 58
embodied play 51, 71; *see also* sensory play

embodiment development 82–4, 113–16
Embodiment-Projection-Role (EPR) 51, 81, 82; Embodiment stage 82–4, 88; group sessions 88–94; Projective stage 85–6, 88; Role stage 86–8
emotional dysregulation, and puppets 106–7
emotional effects of domestic violence 66, 67
emotional engagement 158
emotional issues, and touchstone stories 10–13
empathy 7, 24
empowerment 72, 88
environment: embodying 113–16; home 185–6, 187; natural 115, 116–17
EPR *see* Embodiment-Projection-Role (EPR)
equipment *see* play materials
extended consciousness 35
eye-contact, and puppets 101

fear: and the brain 181; of dogs 39; of needles 59–60; and puppets 99–100
feel good cards 70
fetal alcohol syndrome 179–80
Field, Tiffany 167
focused play therapy 183
free-play 86
Freud, Sigmund 34, 68

games: as distraction 58; *see also* activities
Gantt, L. 19
Gateway, C. 187
Gerhardt, S. 114
Goldilocks and the Three Bears group activity 93–4
Green, E. 25
Greenspan, Stanley 133
grooming 21
grounded cognition theory 114–15
group rules 90, 108–9, 168–9
group sessions: discipline 90, 108–9, 168–9; domestic violence 69–70; multiple disabilities 133, 140–3; NDP/EPR 88–94; outdoor 118–26; psycheducation 104, 105; puppets 104, 108–9; Theraplay 167–74
Group Theraplay 163–74; and brain research 165–6; sessions 167–74; and touch research 166–7
guided imagery 58

Hall, T. M. 102
Hambrick, E. 182
Harter, S. 29–30, 35–6, 37, 41
helping hand activity 70
hierarchy of needs model 23–5, *24*
home environment 185–6, 187
Horley, E. 87
hormones 150, 165, 166, 181–2
Horner, G. 180
hospitals 47–61; developmental play 49–52; distraction techniques 55–8; individual referrals 59–60; play preparation 52–5; post-procedural play 58–9; recreational play 48–9, 50; special dreams 55, 56, 57
'Huge Bag of Worries, The' 69
hypothalamus 180, 181

imagery, guided 58
imaginative play 124–6; *see also* pretend play
immersion 31–2, 33
improvisation 86
individual interventions: domestic violence 70–4; hospital play 59–60; *see also* case studies; therapeutic touchstone
intake process 8–9, 12, 183–5
intellectual disabilities 130–43; developing sense of self 135–9; group sessions 133, 140–3; psychotherapy 133–4; therapeutic play 132–3; *see also Parent Learn to Play* program
intensity, of play 115–16
interactional skills 135–9
International Journal of Play 2
intrusive memories 21
Ironside, Virginia 69
I-self and Me-self 29–30, 36, 41, 42

James, B. 183
James, William 29, 35, 36
Jernberg, Ann 163, 166
Jung, C. G. 34

kangaroo care 167

language difficulties 99–100, 134–5
lateral prefrontal cortex 40
learned feedback loops 39–40
Learn to Play program 153; *see also Parent Learn to Play* program
Lester, S. 114

Index

Levels of Consciousness model 36–7
limbic system 18, 166, 180, 189
local support networks 70

McGee, C. 72
magic potions activity 122–3
Maiello, Suzanne 140
Martinez, H. 167
masks 70, 87
Maslow, Abraham 23–5, *24*
massage 84, 167, 188, 189, **190**, 195
mastery, and puppets 100
matching ribbons activity 120
materials *see* play materials
medical procedures: play preparation 52–5; post-procedural play 58–9
medulla 180
memory 16, 18–19, 21, 40, 116, 123
metaplay **155**, 158
midbrain 180, 189
mindsight 37, 44
miniature characters 10, 22–3, 40–4
mirror neuron system 139
mobile play kits 71–2
movement: and multiple disabilities 140–1; NDP/EPR 84; outdoor play 124–6; Theraplay 166; and trauma 188, 189
multiple disabilities 130–43; developing sense of self 135–9; group sessions 133, 140–3; psychotherapy 133–4; therapeutic play 132–3
music 55, 166, 188, 189, 195

Naber, F. 151
narratives, play 154, **155**, **156**; *see also* stories
natural environments 115, 116–17
NDP *see* Neuro-Dramatic-Play (NDP)
needle phobias 59–60
neglect 65, 75, 114, 182, 186; effects on brain 65, 181, 184, 188–9
neural plasticity 114
Neuro-Dramatic-Play (NDP) 81–4, 88–94
Neurosequential Model of Therapeutics (NMT) 166, 183–5, 188–96, **190–4**
neurotransmitters 180–1
Nicholson, B. 167
'Nifflenoo called Nevermind' 70
NMT *see* Neurosequential Model of Therapeutics (NMT)

non-directive play therapy 32, 68, 72; *see also* child-centred play therapy
non-verbal communication 101, 134–5, 137–9
Norrie McCain, N. 149

object substitution **156**, 159
O'Connor, K. J. 35
Ogden, Pat 136
one to one interventions: domestic violence 70–4; hospital play 59–60; *see also* case studies; therapeutic touchstone
open access play 68
opioids 150
outdoor play 113, 115, 116–27; activities 119–26; resources 117–18; running sessions 119–20; safety 117
oxytocin 150

Panksepp, Jaak 132
parental sensitivity 150–1
parental separation, and puppets 104, 105
parent-child play sessions 171–4; *see also* Parent Learn to Play program
parent-child relationships 149–51; *see also* attachment
Parent Learn to Play program 151–61, **155–7**
Parker, L . 167
Peled, E. 69
perinatal care 180
Perry, Bruce 166, 180–1, 182, 184, 185, 188
phobias 40; needle 59–60
physical abuse 66, 83, 182
physical effects of domestic violence 66, *67*
physical play 83
Piaget, Jean 72
play circles 71
play development 51, 132–3, 152, 153–4, **154–7**
play materials: domestic violence interventions 69–70, 71–2; in hospitals 49; making puppets 109; NDP/EPR groupwork 85–6, 87, 89; outdoor play 117–18, 124–5
playrooms: domestic violence interventions 71; hospitals 49
play scripts 154, **155**, **156**; *see also* stories

play skills 51, 132–3, 152, 153–4, 155–7
Play Therapy Dimensions Model 30–4, 31, 38
pons 180
positive framing 55, 61
Positive Psychology 81
post-procedural play 58–9
PRACTICE 187–8
praising 152
pretend play 51, 152–3, 154, 155–7
preventative interventions 68–9, 75, 107, 108
pre-verbal memories 16
Projection *see* Embodiment-Projection-Role (EPR)
projective play 22, 71, 85
proprioception 124
proto-self 35
psycheducation: and puppets 104–6; and touchstone stories 21
psychotherapy 133–4
puppets 97–110; children's use of 98–101; in hospitals 52–4, 54, 59; practitioner use of 101–9; psycheducation 104–6; and touchstone stories 22; types of 109–10
puzzles, as distraction 58

rainbows group activity 91–2
recreational play, in hospitals 48–9, 50
relationship development 91, 140–1; *see also* Parent Learn to Play program
relationships, parent-child 149–51; *see also* attachment
relaxation exercises 186, 188; *see also* massage
repetition 143, 157, 186, 188–9
resilience 25, 68
resources *see* play materials
Rey, E. 167
rhythm: and multiple disabilities 138, 140–1; NDP/EPR 82, 83, 84; Theraplay 166
Rogers, Carl 7, 24
Role *see* Embodiment-Projection-Role (EPR)
role play 51, 71, 86–7, 156
Rubin, Phyllis 163
rules, group 90, 108–9, 168–9
Russell, W. 114

safety: home environment 185; hospital play 49; need to feel safe 20, 24, *24*, 25–6; outdoor play 117
Schore, Allan 137
secure attachment 150–1
self: sense of 135–9; theories of 29–30, 35–6, 41, 42; *see also* consciousness
self-initiation of play 158
self-regulation 114, 164, 166, 186–7
sense of self 135–9
sensitive stress response 114
sensory development 113–14, 122
Sensory Mapping 119–23
sensory play 92, 94, 116, 119–23, 124–6, 133
sequence, ability to 19
serious case reviews 65
sexual abuse 66, 83, 104, 182
Siegel, Daniel 37, 39–40, 139
singing 55, 83, 186
smell, sense of 123
social context of play 152
social effects of domestic violence 66, 67
social skills 88–9, 109, 168, 174
somatic theory 113–16
sound mapping activity 121–2
special dreams 55, 56, 57
Stagnitti, Karen 133
star charts 58
Steele, W. 185
stories: in children's play 85, 86, 155–7; domestic violence interventions 16, 69, 70; and puppets 107–8; *see also* therapeutic touchstone
Strange Situation procedure 150
stress 114, 150, 181–2
stress hormones 150, 165, 181–2
structured play timetable, in hospitals 49, 50
Sunderland, Margot 70, 108, 149–50, 158
superhero picnics activity 58–9
supervision 186
support networks 70
surgery: play preparation 52–5; post-procedural play 58–9
Symbolic and Imaginative Play Developmental Checklist (SIP-DC) 154
symbolic clients, puppets as 102–3, 109–10
Symbolic Play Scale 154

synapses 180–1
Szalavitz, M. 180–1, 185

talking about play **155**, 158
talking stick activity 122
teenagers 58, 88–9
Test of Pretend Play 157
Thayer, T. 167
Theoretical Integration 30
therapeutic touchstone 7–26; children with adjustment issues 13–15; children with complex histories 17, 20–1; children with emotional issues 10–13; and need to feel safe 20, 24, *24*, 25–6; telling the stories 9–10, 22–3; writing the stories 15–20
Theraplay 163–74, 187, 189, 190, **191, 194;** and brain research 165–6; sessions 167–74; and touch research 166–7
Tinnin, L. W. 19
touch 83–4, 166–7, 189, **190**
touchstone, therapeutic *see* therapeutic touchstone
touch toys 58
toys: attributing properties 152, **156**; in hospitals 49; touch toys 58; *see also* dolls; puppets
transitional objects 84
trauma: effects on brain 18–19, 181, 182–3; and touchstone stories 16, 21

Trauma Focused Cognitive Behavioural Therapy (TF CBT) 187–8
trauma informed interventions 183–5, 188–96, **190–4**
Tregay, Janine 163
Trevarthen, Colwyn 136
trust 8

unconditional positive regard 7, 24
unhelpful thoughts 104, 105
Upton, Jason 139

Van der Kolk, B. A. 18
van IJzendoorn, M. 150–1
verbal communication: language difficulties 99–100, 134–5; and puppets 101
visual impairment 134
visualisation 58, 123–4
Vygotsky, Lev 152

Winnicott, D. W. 84
Woltmann, A. G. 100
woodland 116
working memory 40
worries, and puppets 99–100
worry dolls 69–70

yoga 188, 189

Zelazo, P. D. 36–7